TOTAL GLOW

Dr. Rona's Unbeatable Health Program

by Luanne Rona, M.D.

Incorporating
Nutrition, Exercise, Relaxation

The material presented in this book is intended to help you become more knowledgeable about your health, and to encourage you to take care of your body and mind. In no way is it intended for use as a diagnosis or prescription. You are encouraged to cooperate with your physician. Use of any information for yourself is your constitutional right, but the author and publisher assume no responsibility.

© Copyright 1978 by Luanne Rona, M.D.

ISBN: 0-913864-28-5

Library of Congress Catalog No. 78-62657

All rights reserved. No part of this book, except for brief passages in articles and reviews that refer to both author and publisher, may be reproduced in any form without written permission from the publisher.

Published By: Enterprise Publishing Co., Inc.
1300 Market Street
Wilmington, DE 19801

*True enjoyment comes from
activity of the mind and exercise of the body;
the two are ever united.*
—**Humboldt**

Acknowledgements

I would like to thank the entire staff of Enterprise Publishing Company and its related companies for their interest, support, and suggestions; especially Joe Pasquini, Margaret Buchanan, and T. N. Peterson, for their comments. For suggestions in the area of recipes, I thank Maggie Hickson, my wonderful friend and gourmet cooking partner, Carol Overman, and especially Jan Seely who spent many hours working with me, laboring over these efforts.

I want to give my deepest appreciation to Beverly Kirby, editor for Enterprise Publishing Co., who worked and struggled with me, and became a health believer in the process. Her help was invaluable and will always be remembered.

*To Nick
Whose Love Of Life Is A
Constant Source Of
Inspiration*

Contents

Foreword *by Ted Nicholas* xiv
Preface *by Dwight L. McKee, M.D.* xviii

Day 1
Overview: What the Total Glow Program Means to You
    Prevention... 1
    The Integration of the Individual 1
    Psychosomatic Illnesses............................... 2
    The Elements of the Total Approach 3
    Cancer Research 3
    The Need for Physical Activity 4
    The Need for Relaxation............................... 6
    "The Greatest Truths Are Often The Simplest" 8
    The Federal Drug Administration's Role................ 9
    Life Expectancy 10

The Essentials
    How the Total Glow Program Works................... 13
    Exercise — Why We Need It.......................... 15
    Meditation — How to Do It.......................... 19
    Nutrition — Suggestions for Improvement.............. 22
    An Historical Look at Food 25
    A Psychological Look at Food 25

The Total Glow Health Questionnaire
    A Self-test to Determine Your Physical and
    Emotional Health 27
    Answers and Discussions 29

Day 2
The Importance of Relaxation
    How Your Personality Affects Your Health 39
    Case History I (Benefits of Spot Meditation)............ 40

Contents

Case History II (One Businessman's Story) 41
Case History III (A Young Executive's Experience) 42
The Four Levels of Brain Wave Activity 43
Physiological Effects of Meditation................... 45
Second Day's Meditation Instructions.................. 46
Some Interesting Variations 48
Questions and Answers About Meditation............... 49

Exercise — It's Easier Than You Think
Why Vigorous Exercise Isn't Necessary................. 57
Dietary Habits.. 58
How to Turn Everyday Chores Into Exercise 60
Exercises to Help Your Back
    The Cobra...................................... 62
    Elephant Walk.................................. 63
    Shoulder Tension Reliever...................... 64
    Arm Swings..................................... 65
Exercises for Your Stomach, Waist and Abdomen
    Inverted Bend.................................. 66
    Sledge Hammer.................................. 67
    The Half Locust 68
    The Bow 69
    The Triangle 70
    The Plough 71
    Sit Ups With a Chair 72
    Semi Sit Ups................................... 73
    The Crab....................................... 73
    Scissor Kicks.................................. 74
    Rib Cage Lifts................................. 75
Exercises for Your Legs
    Arc Angels..................................... 76
    The Hamstring Stretch 77
    The Swashbuckler............................... 78
    Bottom Lifts................................... 79
    Rockettes Kicks 80
    Toe Raises..................................... 81
Exercises for Specific Areas
    Double Chin Chasers............................ 82
    Swing Strengtheners 83
    Pre-jogging Stretch 84
    Thigh Trimmers................................. 85

Contents

    Knee Pull Ups 85
Aerobics
    Jogging 87
    Cycling 89
    Swimming 90
    Walking 91
    Roving and Hiking 92

Day 3
Eating For Your Health and Happiness
    What is Junk Food? 93
    Human Evolution and Food 93
    How Our Views About Food Can Hurt Us 94
    How to Clear Up Misconceptions About Dieting . 95
    Desireable Weights for Men, Women and Children 96
    Your Metabolism and What It Means 96
    How to Listen to Your Body 100
    "What I Eat" Charts 101
    Diet Awareness Questionnaire 105
    Steps to Healthier Eating 108
    How to Get More Nutrition from the Food You Eat 113
    A Critical Look at Sugar — Some Startling Facts
    You Probably Didn't Know 114
    Sugar Awareness Chart 117
    A Clearer Understanding of Salt 117
    Salt Awareness Chart 119

Additives and Preservatives in Your Life
    Do They Belong There? 120
    BHT/BHA 121
    Some Substances Found in an
    Ordinary Carton of Ice Cream 122
    The Organs of Detoxification 122
    What Medical Tests Can't Tell You 123
    Junk Food Addicts - The Effects on Our Children 123
    Insecticides 125
    Are You a Food Faddist? 128
    Helping Your Body Do Its Job 129
    Your Skin — And How to Care for It 130
        Saunas 132
        Dry Brush Massage 132

Contents

    Oil Massage 134
    Your Liver and Your Life 134
    Don't Blame the Doctors if They Don't Know 135
    Nutrition and Having a Baby...................... 137
    The Role of the Father 139
    The Well-Fed Baby 139
    The Possible Causes of Cancer.................... 140
    How to Protect Yourself from Cancer............... 143

Food Supplements
    Why We Need Them 144
    Which Ones We Need........................... 145
    Dr. Rona's Suggestions 147
    Mineral Guide................................. 153
    The Three Inexpensive Steps to Better Health......... 155
    Vitamin Toxicity............................... 155

Water — A Frightening Awakening
    How Does Your City Rate in Safe Water?............. 156
    Some Predictions and Alternatives 158

The Subject of Nitrates and Nitrites 158

Pet Nutrition...................................... 159
    Supplementing a Pet's Diet 160

Day 4
Implementing the Plan
    Suggestions for Achieving Total Glow................ 161
    The Total Glow Health Policy..................... 164
    Special Considerations.......................... 165
        The Popcorn Problem 165
        The Hot Fudge Sundae Solution 166

Guidelines — How to Do It
    Gradual Approach............................. 167
    Fresh Fruits................................... 167
    Dried Fruits................................... 168
    New Experiences With Breads..................... 168
    Yogurt.. 169
    The Natural Food Dinner Party.................... 169

Contents

Fruit and Vegetable Juices 169
Coffee Substitutes................................. 170
Brown Rice.. 171
Your Water Supply 171
Pasta Products.................................... 171
Sweet Substitutes 171
Legumes 172
Cookware and Utensils 172

Summary of the Total Glow Program
One More Look at Meditation...................... 173
Working Exercise Into Your Life................... 174
Helping Your Family to Be Happier and Healthier 175

Self Tests
Weight/Body Shape/Muscle Tone 177
Nutrition/Diet..................................... 180
Meditation/Relaxation 181
The Total Glow Health Barometer 183

Introduction to the Recipes
Breakfast Recipes 188
Sandwich/Luncheon Recipes....................... 193
Snack Recipes..................................... 195
Dip and Condiment Recipes 196
Soup Recipes...................................... 201
Salad and Dressing Recipes 206
Vegetable Recipes................................. 208
Main Dish Recipes................................. 214
Bread Recipes 231
Dessert Recipes................................... 234
Total Glow Party Buffet Menu and Recipes 244
Seven-day Menu Plan.............................. 248

Supplemental Readings
Converting Your Recipes.......................... 251
How to Grow Your Own Sprouts 253
Some Helpful Household Utensils.................. 253

Bibliography 255

Contents

Suggested Readings.............................. 257
Index... 261
Index to the Recipes............................. 264

Foreword

Until the last couple of years, my main concerns in life were business interests and my writing career. Since then, they've included an intense involvement in better health.

Boy, was I suffering from some false assumptions! After work every day, I used to jog several miles, or play a couple hours of tennis, which I still do. I took some vitamin supplements and ate what I considered to be a pretty good diet—you know, lots of steak, salads, fruits, some (overcooked) vegetables, but also plenty of junk foods and sweets. I never really paid close attention to my diet. I had always received a "very good" bill of health from my annual physical check-ups. I really made sure I saw a physician for a total check at least once a year, in addition to visits for minor complaints. But in a subtle way, I began noticing some changes in my overall health.

I wasn't sick, but just started feeling tired sooner each day. By early evening, I was quite exhausted. I just didn't have the energy to do all the things I wanted to do. I had to push myself to make social plans in the evenings. Sometimes what could be relaxation turned into a chore.

I really didn't enjoy that feeling of weariness which seemed to be gradually increasing to include more of the day. At that point in my life, I was accomplishing (by most standards) several times the things most people did. But I still sensed that something was wrong. And I knew it was not merely the fact that I had passed the age of forty.

I decided to really make some personal changes in my life and get even more serious about practicing better health habits. I wanted to feel better, have more energy, and improve the overall quality of living. I began to get deeper into more research in the major areas of preventive health.

After many years of struggling with a smoking habit, I finally overcame the addiction. This was most difficult for me, but a friend who died of lung cancer in her early forties really helped scare me into the final decision to quit. After I became aware of Dr. Rona's work in a total approach to health, I volunteered to help test and share the benefits of the many nutritional recipes. From that point on, the biggest change I underwent was in my diet. But I approached the whole idea of changing food and know it has its benefits. The preparation of meals is a fun project. I treated food shopping and searching for special ingredients and cooking as a hobby, which fortunately resulted in the most rewarding benefits for me: a healthy, happier life.

While this book was being written, I was among the fortunate people who got to try the recipes and vote on which ones should be included in the book. I also tried all the exercises and have been enjoying meditation for some time. It seems almost unbelievable now, but at first I had a negative image of nutritious foods. I just didn't think they would taste good, for some reason. Happily, I was wrong.

I also really considered people somewhat "nutty" who went overboard in this area. I thought that health food buyers tended to be eccentrics with their gurus, incense, sandals, beards, beads, etc. But I gained a lot of pleasure from learning about many new things, like trying new vegetables, grains, and sprouts that I'd never tasted before. I also took a course on nutrition and gained the qualifications of a certified nutritionist, just so I could learn more about health. Most of what I've learned, however, Dr. Rona has taught me.

This book contains all she has taught me and more. Her purpose is not to make claims of miraculous cures for disease. However, I've personally met some people recently who have had gravely serious illnesses including arthritis, heart disease, and terminal cancer, who have completely recovered after giving up on drugs and other treatments and going on a sound nutritional health program. Others have found relief from asthma, diverticulosis, psoriasis, and other similar diseases of the liver, prostate, pancreas, and headaches, backaches, all through the natural approach to life. All of this will be revealed to you in this book.

One of the most amazing things to me has been the discovery that most physicians know little or nothing about nutrition. Almost no nutritional training is given in medical schools. Fortunately, some doctors are beginning to show an interest in this vitally important area. When the medical profession becomes more aware of this, perhaps the same type of fine results such as have occurred in crisis medicine and with the treatment of illness will be evidenced in the enormously important area of prevention.

Presently, I'm busy enjoying fresh, pure foods, fresh juices, pure water, exercising, and meditating, and feeling better than I've ever felt in my life. This enables me to keep up with an active business, athletic, and social life. I'm gratified that you have chosen to read this book, for I know how much you will gain from it.

Before writing this book, Dr. Rona originally had scheduled a series of seminars on another subject. I was so pleased when she decided to drop those to write this book. She realized that was a far more important, although difficult, project to undertake because there was no complete and integrated book available to combine the three life-serving areas of nutrition, exercise, and relaxation, plus a common-sense psychological approach.

The author has successfully tied together the most vital area which, when practiced, will result in a person whose mind and body is an integrated whole. I know from personal experience that the information in this book can entirely change your life, both spiritually and physically from within.

I hope you enjoy yourself as much as I have on your journey to inner peace and outer radiance, which is "Total Glow." As Dr. Rona says, "You deserve every bit of it, and you *can* have it."

Ted Nicholas

Preface

I am very excited about this book. Until now, there haven't been any books on health improvement which provide a holistic approach. There are countless (and often contradictory) books on nutrition, many on exercise, and just as many covering the areas of mental attitude and positive thinking. Dr. Rona's book, however, is the first one which integrates nutrition and exercise with mental and emotional health improvement techniques in a sensible, workable program.

Some of the best-selling books in recent years have been on the subject of running. Why the sudden explosive interest in this type of exercise? My guess is that so many people in America feel *bad,* that they are turning to anything which makes them feel better. Running stimulates and strengthens the adrenal glands which are the primary sources of biological substances which provide us with a sense of energy, alertness, and well-being. They are also the prime target of stress.

Refined sugar and caffeine, upon which so many Americans depend to "get them started" and "keep them going," compound the assault on the adrenal glands, until a state of nearly constant fatigue is reached. This is lifted only by regular doses of these stimulants. Overstressed, malnourished, suffering from exercise- and sunlight-deficiencies, Americans have become a nation of addicts. We are addicted to sugar, caffeine, alcohol, nicotine, and television.

The dramatic discoveries of methods to control infectious disease over the last four decades has spawned the huge industry of modern allopathic medicine. With the growth of "crisis care," people gradually turned over the responsibility for their health to the medical profession. In turn, they turned their responsibility for their food and self-medication to Madison Avenue advertising and the food industry. Now we see that we have traded the scourge of infectious disease for the degenerative ones.

Modern medicine is powerless in the face of the rapidly advancing modern plagues of heart disease, cancer, diabetes, and arthritis. People are beginning to realize that prevention of these diseases lies in their lifestyles. Professor Wrba, head of the Austrian Cancer Institute, stated to the Austrian Government that he could cut the incidence of cancer by 50% in that country within two years, if they could change the diet of the entire nation. The dietary changes he recommended are *precisely those outlined in this book.*

We are beginning to see that some high-level decisions, made thirty years ago on the basis of scientific evidence available at that time, were wrong. Putting nitrate, potassium, phosphorus (surplus chemicals from World War II explosives industries) in the soil did stimulate and increase agricultural production, but they also destroyed the delicate ecological balance of micro-organisms in the topsoil, and depleted it. Hence, our food supply of the essential trace minerals, such as manganese, chromium, zinc, cobalt, and selenium, has been depleted. Their significance in metabolism was not yet recognized when the industrial movement in agriculture came about. Likewise, the idea that we could improve on nature by removing the germ and the bran from wheat and replacing these things with several synthetic B vitamins (to make "enriched" white flour) has proved fallacious.

People are becoming more aware that it is foolish to leave decisions about the quality and source of food to people who have large profit motives involved. It is interesting to note that not ONE of the high level executives of the second largest soft drink company in the world consumes the beverage upon which that company was founded. Perhaps they know something that we don't know.

The proliferation of natural food stores (here again, avoid the large chains which market expensive vitamin and mineral supplements primarily, and look for ones dedicated to providing organic produce whenever possible, along with whole grains, beans, nuts, and seeds in bulk), the interest in exercise and holistic health centers are encouraging signs that Americans are ready to take more responsibility for their own nutrition, health, and well-being.

As Associate Medical Director of one of the few holistic health centers in New England, I see the positive benefits of natural foods, nutrition, exercise, and relaxation on a daily basis—the building blocks of Dr. Rona's TOTAL GLOW program. In the three years since our clinic has been in operation, interest has grown to such an extent that our waiting list for appointments will take a year to accommodate! Until now, we have not had an adequate self-help manual for such people to begin incorporating health-building practices into their lifestyles, especially one that combines all aspects of health which we emphasize in holistic health care. I am truly grateful to Dr. Rona for providing us with this book.

May Health and Peace be with you all,
Dwight L. McKee, M.D.

Day 1
Introduction: An Overview

Prevention
The Integration of the Individual

Never before in history has the importance of prevention been more crucial than it is today. From the prevention of nuclear warfare, to putting a stop to the sufferings of the poor, to curing the ills of those with terrible diseases such as cancer, the key word is *prevention*.

We are managing to handle the crises in medicine, but the underlying cure is through preventing the disease from ever starting. If only the primary symptoms of an illness are treated, how long can the patchwork last, especially when the *cause* may go unrecognized?

There are many topics I would like to write about, but after surveying the world around me, I found the most urgent and compelling subject to be that of total health. It is an enjoyable subject, since treating and helping people has been my endeavor and my joy since childhood.

The background for my theory of total health came from my work as a psychiatrist, where I have helped many people deal with the tensions and stresses of everyday living. For many years, I found that emotional upsets lead to physical troubles. It became apparent to me at the same time that a person who was in less-than-satisfactory physical condition could not make progress as rapidly as those who were healthier. It is amazing how many people try to separate themselves into physical and mental halves.

It was then that the vast importance of treating an individual as a mental and physical unit was realized. To concentrate on a person's emotional state at the expense of their physical well-being was, in effect, to deny the person as a total, integrated human being. A person consists of a body *and* a mind, and the definition does not apply to one without the other.

My definition of "Total Glow," the title of this book, is: A state of optimal health that reflects an inner peace and an outward radiance. I do not believe that one can be achieved to the exclusion of the other.

Unfortunately, it has been somewhat common in medical and philosophical circles to deny that these two elements of a person are connected in anything but the slightest way. Most religions, both Western and Eastern, seek to deny what is human and strive for an ideal, almost body-less existence. Poets, writers, and philosophers have grappled with their desire to escape from the sordid physical world for centuries. The medical profession has been repeatedly accused of ignoring the "person" while treating the "ailment."

All of these examples are indications of our culture's unwillingness to accept ourselves as physical and mental units, both of which are attempting to function harmoniously.

Psychosomatic Illness

When the physical and mental demands people make upon themselves get out of kilter, something usually suffers. Psychosomatic diseases are one way in which the body tells the mind to "STOP!" Similarly, the mind tells the body what to do in common situations. For example, when we become angry, tense, or frightened, our fists clench, palms sweat, brows furrow, pupils dilate, and muscles clamp in preparation for fight or flight. This fight-or-flight phenomenon is an automatic response wherein the organism (our body) mobilizes itself when encountered by a stressful situation. It prepares itself for performance; either to confront or retreat from danger.

Due to the inescapable connection and interaction between mind and body then, it is much more effective to treat an individual as an integrated human being, rather than by ignoring physical ailments and treating emotional problems exclusively.

The self-improvement program described in this book is the outcome of this theory, when put into practice. As a medical doctor, I saw a great need for a method through which people could improve their physical appearance, their health, and their emotional outlook on life *all at the same time*. This book is the result of years of personal research into the areas of relaxation, nutrition, exercise, and psychology.

It has often been said that a person can diet religiously in an effort to lose weight, but that these endeavors will probably be of little long-term value if the diet is not followed with exercise. In the same way, people seeking to improve their physical appearances will have little long-lasting success if they are not relaxed, rested, and healthy underneath the exterior layer.

The Elements of the Total Approach

So the most important element in this self-improvement program is the integration of the individual and the *total approach* to the entire physical and emotional unit. The three major techniques are:
  (1) a nutritional approach to diet, with the gradual development of healthier eating habits,
  (2) exercise, starting off slowly and working up to the most beneficial exercises,
  (3) self-relaxation, a technique that may be practiced as often as desired.

The most powerful element of all is *YOU*. These three techniques can lead to a glowing life (inside and out—that's Total Glow!), but it is up to you to do it. Let your zest for life make itself apparent. Start saying to yourself that you are unique in all the world, and that you have a right to be the happiest, healthiest person alive. You have a purpose. As the saying goes, "You are extraordinary." Begin to rid yourself of negative slogans, which are the outgrowths of negative philosophies which tell you your life is meaningless. Stop saying, "I'm helpless," "I can't do anything about it," and "I don't deserve it." Leave those debates to others who want to stay entrenched in their misery.

Cancer Research

Keeping this premise in mind, let us consider the subject of food. More and more is being written today about the effects of chemical additives in food on our bodies and minds, and, conversely, about the ravages of accumulated stress and tension. It is common knowledge that certain dietary deficiencies and abuses may cause cancer, high blood pressure, and even hyperactivity in children.[1]

> *"Salt aggravates high blood pressure. Sugar may bring about diabetes. Beef and butter clog the arteries, leading to heart attacks. The rich and abundant U.S. diet has recently been linked to a growing number of serious illnesses, and the worst may be to come. For researchers are now becoming convinced that the foods Americans put on their tables play a major part in the most frightening disease of all–cancer.*
>
> *"The link between diet and cancer has become a political issue. In widely publicized hearings last month, Sen. George McGovern and his subcommittee on nutrition cited evidence*

---

[1]Benjamin F. Feingold, M.D., *Why Your Child is Hyperactive* (New York: Random House, 1975).

that half of all cases of cancer are related to diet. McGovern criticized National Cancer Institute officials for spending only $16 million of their current $876 million budget to study the role of nutrition in cancer, while consuming $100 million in the still-fruitless search for cancer-causing viruses.

"The strongest clues to the role of diet in cancer come from epidemiological studies of population groups. The highest rates of bowel cancer, for example, occur in countries with the highest consumption of beef, which is rich in animal fats."[2]

"Speaking before the Senate nutrition subcommittee, research scientists said the cancer war, officially declared in 1970 and lavishly funded since then, has hunted unsuccessfully for cures while ignoring prevention related to nutritional and environmental activities. The witnesses noted that the National Cancer Institute budget has increased fourfold in seven years to more than $800 million; but cancer research 'now faces a crisis of credibility,' Dr. Theodore Cooper, dean of Cornell University Medical College said.

"A top cancer researcher at Harvard Medical School said there is a traditional emphasis on treating diseases rather than preventing them, and that in 1976 just 19 of the country's 114 medical schools required nutrition courses."[3]

It appears to be a vicious cycle which compounds upon itself and ultimately damages our health.

The Need for Physical Activity

The public is also probably all too well aware of the importance of exercise to physical well-being; so aware that too many of us are turned off by the more rigorous approach. Surprisingly, research is finding that exercise need not be all that strenuous to be of benefit, and that even our intelligence quotients may rise with regular exercise, because of the increased supply of oxygen to the brain.

It is the goal of my program to help you realize the necessity of tying these three areas together into a comprehensive program whereby you may embark upon a course of self-improvement which will enhance not only your physical appearance, but your emotional outlook as well.

Each of you probably knows one or two very lucky people who have the self-discipline to carry out a precise diet/exercise/relaxation pro-

---

[2]Newsweek, "Cancer and Our Diet." July 24, 1978.

[3]*The Wall Street Journal,* "The War on Cancer." June 13, 1978.

gram through the years. These are the very people you often meet who appear to be virtually bubbling over with enthusiasm, vitality, ambition, good looks, and health. The attainment of this "glow of health" is the goal of this program, and can be your goal, too. Statistics show, however, that a good forty percent of the adult population of the United States is overweight, or similarly unhealthy in some way. I would estimate that more people are subclinically unhealthy than any statistics can show. Physicians are hearing the statement, "I've never been sick—how can this be happening to me?" more often.

Medical research has shown that the problems caused by inattention to one's health can in many cases be reversed or, at the very least, slowed down with proper care. Naturally, it is much easier to become fit and stay fit throughout life, but the statistics mentioned earlier reveal that an overwhelming proportion of people are not only less than physically fit, but are, quite frankly, in deplorable shape. Among the most frequent victims of self-neglect are business and professional people.

Delaney Kiphuth, Yale University's Director of Athletics, Physical Education, and Recreation, said in a recent interview in a national magazine,

"People tend to get into a 'lazy state' during the 20 to 30 (age) period.... There's no question about that–they're preoccupied in getting started in their life's work."

Another professor of Physical Education, Dr. David Costill of Ball State University, reiterated Kiphuth's statement when he said,

"Probably the most important years are between 25 and 35. It's during those years that a lot of atherosclerosis* seems to start. Most people at that time ... are quite involved in occupations and careers and never do really establish a pattern of regular physical activity.... We have seen a number of men and women who have been totally inactive for twenty to thirty years.... It's just unbelievable how little they have done."

Years ago, there was little need for physical fitness programs. People did their laundry by hand, scrubbed floors on their knees, chopped their own wood, built their own houses and barns, and essentially did all the physical work that "modern conveniences" perform today. We now live in an age when most adults spend the majority of their waking lives sitting down. Certainly, their minds are quite active, but bodies seem to have become a necessary inconvenience.

The result of this inactivity is visible every day. Usually the rationalization people make for neglecting themselves is the oft-

---

*A thickening and loss of elasticity in the walls of the arteries with the formation of fatty deposits.

repeated statement: "I'm too busy." It seems as if we are so busy getting on with our careers or with raising our families that there is a tendency to neglect the most important asset we own—ourselves. Or, more specifically, our health.

In addition to the ultimate importance of regular physical activity, some of the additional responsibility we must accept is that for our own diets. Nutrition is currently an emotion-packed controversial issue, and the debate will probably continue for many years to come. It is the intention of this book, however, to present some practical, sensible guidelines for improvement in this area.

It has been proved many times that certain substances added in the processing of food and other products for consumption are harmful to the human body. Greater numbers of these substances are being discovered everyday, and it is likely that this will continue. It is a fundamental contention of mine that overly processed foods are unhealthy and that there are numerous delicious, inexpensive alternatives. Everyone can easily and comfortably live without all the chemical additives while at the same time be greatly improving their health.

The Need for Relaxation

In addition to an excellent program of proper nutrition and exercise, the value and absolute importance of a calm, relaxed state of mind must be emphasized. It cannot be denied that a person is unable to improve their physical appearance to a great extent if their emotions are in turmoil or distress. The opposite is also true; if your body is weakened by pain or burdened with excess weight or chemical toxins, your mental picture cannot be too bright, either.

There are many things that contribute to the disintegration of the individual in our rapidly changing society. The major one is stress; that tension which works on the mind and body until something eventually has to give. Psychosomatic illness is one way in which "something gives." These are real, physical illnesses (and anyone who has had an ulcer can attest to that), but they are caused by stress. Ulcers, tension headaches, spastic colon, reactive hypertension, insomnia, some skin disorders, and even alcoholism and drug dependence are examples of psychosomatic, stress-related illnesses.

In the most primitive form, this is how the body signals the mind that something is wrong with the way it is dealing with stress. It is when this anxious state of mind continues unremittingly for long periods of time that the body simply rebels and produces a physical impairment or dysfunction.

For instance, a doctor will often tell a high blood pressure patient that he must learn to relax. Although this type of advice is probably the best a physician can render, many doctors fall short in the explanation of the ways the patient can *learn* to relax. The patient is then left in a stress-producing quandary, and may turn to methods that promise overnight rewards, or other questionable practices that may only make matters worse in the long run.

Through this program, you can teach yourself one of the oldest and simplest relaxation methods in the world—meditation. This form of meditation is not connected with the esoteric form practiced by many followers today.

When first introduced to the Eastern form of meditation, I found the technique quite valuable, but was somewhat concerned about the promises made and by the necessary adherence to foreign religious beliefs. So, borrowing from the basic technique of meditation, but eliminating all the mystical aspects, a system of self-relaxation was developed.

This new form is centered around you, rather than focused upon an idol or god, and can be learned through the instructions in this book. It isn't necessary to attend a course or study any other materials, though you may wish to do some further readings if you are interested. The instructions are all contained herein, and you can learn it in four easy steps.

This technique is readily adaptable and workable for people of all ages, lifestyles, and beliefs. It will not change or transform you into anything more or less than a relaxed and vital person able to deal with everyday tension and stress in a more constructive manner. Chances are excellent that it will improve your sense of self-esteem, your self-confidence, and your assertiveness.

Meditation will enable you to release built-up tension on a regular basis so that you may get on with your life and the more enjoyable aspects of it. It is not necessary to accept any strange religious beliefs or teachings, since it is merely a practical, no-nonsense approach to self-relaxation, and it is one of the easiest techniques to learn and maintain.

The total program is set up on a four-day approach because I believe that the majority of readers will be results-oriented and busier than most. The four-day approach is a quick, encapsulated presentation of the basic goals of the Total Glow program, and the ways in which you may go about achieving them. It is specifically designed for those people who are intimately involved in their work and homelife, and who have previously been unable to devote extensive amounts of time to self-improvement programs.

In the same vein, the Total Glow program was designed to be an extremely flexible and adaptable one in which each one of you may tailor-make your own schedule to fit your needs and timetable. There isn't a pass-or-fail grading system in the program, and no restrictive time limits are imposed. It is a program through which you progress at your own pace, and realize achievement goals at your own rate.

There are many excellent self-improvement books on the market today dealing with either diet, exercise, or relaxation exclusively, but I believe that improvement in all three areas in conjunction will yield the highest, most satisfying, and most permanent results. Just as you cannot lose weight effectively through dieting alone, so it is that self-improvement efforts in one direction only will not be as effective or all-encompassing. And just as beauty does not come from youth or facial structure alone, so it is that optimum health and vitality cannot be achieved through attention to the physical body exclusively. Inner beauty, and the "glow of health" come from well-tuned bodies and calm, relaxed minds.

It is my personal desire that through this book you will begin a self-improvement program that will result in the realization of both short- and long-term goals, to the eventual betterment of your entire life.

The Total Glow program is not a difficult one to follow. It does not contain a deprivational diet plan where you will feel punished, nor does it contain strenuous exercises that will require special equipment or membership in an exclusive club. Self relaxation, too, is one of the simplest techniques available, and it is exceptionally easy to learn.

The Greatest Truths are Often the Simplest

In this society, a great deal of emphasis has been placed upon physical attractiveness. Many people look upon the old, the infirm, the plain, or the unattractive with views ranging from pity to contempt. To my way of thinking, a person's energy, vitality, and zest for life, and that certain serene inner glow of health, are the true marks of beauty. Through following this program, these qualities can be attained. Give it a try. Remember, it's your life and the best way is to really live it!

I have many pictures and posters surrounding me to remind us of what may seem to be the obvious. One of my favorites is:

"The Greatest Truths are Often the Simplest."

Somehow, those involved in medicine tend to be baffled or frightened by the killing diseases; so much so that we miss what could be some of the *simpler* ways to prevent and alleviate them.

As in psychiatry, the concept of the fundamental importance of self-esteem as the basic requirement for mental health, often was and is still grossly neglected. We get caught in the complexities and seem to lose sight of the obvious.

Penicillin was the wonder drug of the 1940's and steroids were the miraculous advance of the 1950's. Since then, it has been progressing from one drug to another. While gigantic and laudable strides have been made in curing diseases, we have neglected adequately investigating ways to *prevent* them from developing in the first place.

We have become increasingly conditioned to look for a form of magic from doctors and dentists in order that everything will be all right and we will be cured of what ails us. Meanwhile, the physicians and dentists have been busy learning the esoteric information and searching for answers in a similar way.

We have all but forgotten about the nutrients, how to cook to preserve them, and what the demand for fast foods has done to our health in the last twenty-five years. We have slowly become addicted to sugar and salt. With the aim of helping people prepare their foods quickly, or dining out conveniently, many major food industries have left our food with a miniscule portion of the vitamins and minerals we need. Our fast-paced life and lack of interest in exploring our own health potential is another part of the problem.

The Federal Drug Administration's Role

What about the Food and Drug Administration? How many experiments have been conducted to determine the safety of the 5,000 or so chemicals added to our foods? How much have we been told about the possible toxins and long-term effects they may have upon us? Very little!!

Let's look at it this way. Nothing has been written or published to prove that additives *are safe,* even through the short term. If you have left your potato salad out of the refrigerator overnight, would you eat it or serve it to your family? Perhaps you might smell it first to see if it was all right. Even if it smelled and tasted fine, very few people would even think of eating it or serving it to others.

Most of us would throw it away, just to be on the safe side. The rationale would be that it's better to waste a little bit of food than to take a chance on illness or food poisoning.

Additives, preservatives, and other chemical or artificial substances are like the potato salad that has been sitting on the counter all night. There's a *chance* that it won't hurt you, but an even greater chance that it will. Why take the risk when you don't know for certain?

Obviously, the F.D.A. can't be entirely to blame. They are understaffed and overworked (and yet, inexplicably, they have time to investigate health food stores, while only 1% of the farms are inspected for proper insecticide use). It makes one wonder if perhaps there might be some connection between government agencies and certain big businesses responsible for the additives and insecticides.

Getting action on these pressing problems will be up to us. Write your senators and congressmen and demand information about the F.D.A. studies. Don't settle for platitudes such as, "It's okay, don't worry." Don't let yourself be swayed by inadequately researched reports about health foods. In a free society, we have the right to demand that junk food pushers be put out of business! At the very least, you have a right not to die from poisoning at someone else's hands. You have the power to begin to take charge of your life, what you consume, and where it comes from.

The thought may have crossed your mind that I am making a big fuss about nothing. After all, Americans are living longer than ever before. Some people live to be in their late 90's and proudly state that they smoke, drink, and "chase women." But they are individuals. We all have different and unique hereditary make-ups. What might not hurt one person, may mean early death to you.

Yes, our parents are living longer. But if they are over fifty or sixty, they grew up in a healthier nutritional environment than we **did.** Their food came from farms before they started the indiscriminate use of pesticides and artificial fattening agents. More than likely, they had fresh eggs from fertile hens, and vegetables from earth filled with nutrients.

Life Expectancy

Some people are confused by the statistics regarding life expectancy and how it has increased greatly in the past few years. The major reason for this statistical increase is that the death rate *at birth* has declined significantly in the last twenty-five years due to advances in the fields of obstetrics and gynecology. Life expectancy charts are calculated from age at birth. So you can see that by reducing the death rate among newborn infants, the average life expectancy increases accordingly.

Contagious diseases such as tuberculosis, whooping cough, polio, and small pox destroyed many of our ancestors in the primes of their lives. Thanks to the researchers and discoveries of cures of these diseases, they are no longer responsible for taking so many lives. But new diseases, for which there are no known cures at the present time, are taking their places.

Despite intensive research into the two main killing diseases of today (heart trouble and cancer), we are experiencing little advancement, especially in the area of cancer.

One thing is certain, however. A healthy body can better defend itself against disease, including cancer, than can an unhealthy one.

Although there are not any long-established and well-defined studies on which all authorities agree to prove the ways in which you can maintain optimum health, the concepts of the Total Glow program will provide you with many answers and further thought-provoking questions which can lead you to individual ones to discuss with your physician. In addition, you will gain a basic understanding of the road to better—possibly the best—state of health.

Day 1
The Essentials

How the Total Glow Program Works

First days, like all new beginnings, are often filled with anticipation and not a little apprehension. People are often quite occupied with thoughts and questions like:

"Is this really going to work for me?"
and
"Will I measure up?"

Reading this book is a big step, all by itself. You can make a decision to embark upon a course that will lead you to a greater sense of self-esteem through improvement in physical appearance, health, and emotional outlook. It is essential to remember, however, that any self-improvement plan can only be measured by the success of the person undertaking it. It is not the intent of this program to present a grueling formula whereby you will feel deprived, regimented, or self-sacrificing. Instead, it is a program that is designed to be implemented by you in your own special way. Your progress and success is only measurable by you, the individual.

Whether or not this system works for you is, quite frankly, *up to you*. There is a saying that goes, "The reward of the spirit who tries is not the goal, but the exercise." With this in mind, you are encouraged to give yourself the chance to see if this program will help you. Chances are excellent that with the determination to carry through the first initial orientation, this program can and will work for everyone.

The second question—Will I measure up?—simply does not apply to this program. There are many other books where individual goals and time sequences are pre-determined, but there are none of those stringent elements here. You may decide in which directions you wish to go, and the areas in which you want to improve, and chart your own course. You will not find any incredible claims like **"LOSE FIFTY POUNDS IN TWO WEEKS"** in this book.

Time limits are not really recommended since they seem to imply a kind of make-it-or-break ultimatum. These kinds of restrictive goals are too easily missed, and they are often self-defeating, which tends to make you feel even worse. This course is designed to reward you for whatever progress that might be made, rather than arbitrarily establishing universal goals and deadlines, and castigating readers if they do not perform as expected.

The aim is to give you plenty to feel *GOOD* about. It is a laudible accomplishment already that you are reading a book through which you can learn to improve yourself. One area that will enhance increased feelings of self-esteem is meditation.

Meditation

This is one of the easiest and oldest relaxation techniques in the world. It is a quieting, tranquilizing practice, and the results of it will probably surprise you when the time comes to evaluate your progress.

Exercise

These are not those you suffered through in Physical Education class or boot camp. They were specifically chosen for their simplicity and for the rapidity with which they tone and slim the body. They will not make you feel out of breath, or as if your muscles cannot bear another moment of it, like the more traditional exercises would. It is important to start with toning and stretching exercises first, then add jogging, swimming, or walking when you are in better condition. Both types of exercise are necessary.

Diet and Nutrition

This discussion is also fashioned in a gradual method through which you can cleanse your system of accumulated toxins, and begin to realize the many benefits of eating healthful, delicious foods.

The four-day approach is designed so that you may begin the program on the first day that you start reading this book, and by the end of the fourth day's reading, you will be completely familiar with and prepared for the continuation of the Total Glow program. Of course, depending upon each reader's available time, four days may be too short or too lengthy a time to absorb the total program. This, too, is quite flexible.

For instance, if you are planning a vacation shortly where the mainstay of your wardrobe will be swimwear, you can quickly read through the program, start doing all the toning exercises, begin with the nutritional recommendations, and you'll be on your way to an improved appearance in a short time. Vacations are a great time to try meditation, since you have more free time and can arrange it so that you are not interrupted.

On the other hand, if you are planning to once-and-for-all start taking better care of yourself, you might want to go through the program at a slower pace while assimilating the information more thoroughly. It is up to you, and each reader should feel completely free to adapt the program in the way that is best for her/him.

I do recommend a gradual approach. If you expect too much too soon, you can set yourself up for failure and feel much worse. I used to see this happening often with my clients. Now it happens less and less because I am careful to warn them about it. I want you to have this same warning. It is what I call "being gentle to yourself." Try not to blame yourself and throw out the whole program if you make some slips or get out of the routine for a while. Remember that the benefits of the Total Glow program are cumulative. The more relaxed you are, the more healthful foods you eat in place of junk foods, and the more exercise you get will pay off many-fold in the long run.

Exercise: Why We Need It

Exercise is a topic that is frustrating to many people. Mention the word and you are bound to get reactions ranging from disgruntled looks to sighs of resignation. To most people, the word conjures up images of sweatsuits, unsavory atmospheres of public gyms, and strenuous, muscle-wrenching misery. Others will remember with a tinge of guilt, the $39.95 they spent a few years ago on the red polyester warm up suit, or the exercise equipment that now lies gathering dust in the basement.

Actually, in case you haven't noticed, exercise (and the philosophy thereof) has made some grand progress in the past few years. Gone are the days of those miserable jumping jacks, squat thrusts, and push ups. They have since been replaced by simpler things like leisure walking, isometrics, hiking, bicycling, horseback riding, and "spot" toners that are specifically designed *not* to work up a sweat.

Though some physical fitness experts and doctors will still assert that you must get your heart beating rapidly for exercise to do any good, all will agree that this type of activity is not for the beginner, nor for the person who has led a sedentary life for too many years. Jumping rope, jogging, and all other forms of vigorous exercise can come later, *after* you have yourself in good physical condition.

By "good physical condition" I am indicating a person who has exercised regularly four or five times a week for at least six months. Before you embark on a vigorous exercise program, practice the muscle toning exercises and relaxation techniques I've outlined in the book for about two or three months. Always check with your physician before beginning any exercise programs.

After toning the individual muscle groups, you will reduce the possibility of straining or pulling a leg or back muscle when it comes time to try more activity. This also applies to people who are adept at one sport and want to try another that uses an entirely different set of muscles.

At this point, strenuous exercise will do you more harm than good. Chances are that if you attempt to religiously perform a spate of exhaustive exercises from this day forward, you will find yourself in the following predicament within two weeks:

1. Every muscle in your body will be sore.
2. You will find yourself making little excuses for avoiding your daily ritual.
3. You will get discouraged.
4. You will abandon your Great Self-Improvement Plan altogether.

All of this will only serve to make you feel guilty, and even worse—more out of shape than you were when you started. Also, it will make you even more reluctant to ever again attempt an exercise program.

Start slowly. It is not my intent to have you suffering from sore muscles, boredom, a sense of drudgery, or guilt feelings. Exercise is and should be fun, and it makes you feel wonderful, even if you had been feeling tired when you started. Make exercising as enjoyable as possible, even to the point of putting on your favorite records and getting the whole family involved.

The most important thing to remember when you make up your mind to take care of your body is that you must "think" exercise as often as possible. If you can keep the thought in your mind that the exercises you are performing are doing you immeasurable good, even the more difficult ones will be easier. By having exercise on your mind, you can come up with some ingenious methods which can be performed whenever someone else isn't looking—or perhaps, even when they are!

By continually keeping "EXERCISE!" in the back of your mind, you can discover thousands of ways in which to use your body when you otherwise wouldn't. This is another basic element of the Total Glow program. People who are in good physical shape tend to keep themselves that way, simply because it becomes so painfully obvious to them when they fall out-of-shape. The Total Glow program will get you into better physical condition quickly and easily so that you may maintain the consequential feelings of good health and improved appearance.

It isn't too difficult to see the reasons why most adults are in poor physical condition, even though it is sometimes through no fault of their own. They get up and *drive* to work, then *ride* an elevator to their floor, where they *sit* at a desk for eight hours. Lunch might include a *drive* to a restaurant where a cocktail or two and heavy, starchy food is consumed. At the end of the working day, the person *drives* home, *puts the feet up,* while *lounging* over the evening paper. Most then eat the biggest meal of the day, and spend the rest of the evening *lying* or *sitting* on the sofa. Finally, it's off to *bed* to *rest up* for another exhausting day.

It isn't any wonder why most people always feel exhausted! Their minds might have been very active, but their bodies were just sitting around all day doing nothing. A quick survey of businesspeople over thirty in your area will probably tell you that the majority of them are overweight and out of shape. How many pot bellies do you see? Legs were meant for walking, backs for supporting the body, arms for lifting, and bodies for bending and stretching. All the muscles have their own jobs of supporting skeletal structure and internal organs, and almost none of them are kept in shape through sedentary occupations or lifestyles. This is one reason why so many people suddenly pull a muscle or ligament for no apparent reason.

As late as the Turn of the Century, the people in this country had little problem with the illnesses that arise from inactivity. There was laundry to be done by hand, coal to be shoveled, logs to be split, and school to walk to (typically, through three miles in the snow). It was not until the invention of modern household conveniences that we began to get interested in exercise, fat, and the elimination of the latter. It was also around that time that the population became infatuated with the idea of slimness.

I'm not suggesting that you take your laundry to the nearest creek and wash it pioneer-style, nor even that you convert your furnace to coal. There are many ways to work around an inactive lifestyle, and they are easier than you might think.

If you drive to work, consider riding the bus or subway and getting off three or four blocks before your stop. If you must drive, park as far away from your building as you can. Even this short distance is better than door-to-door service, which is tantamount to nothing at all. Also, you will be adding to the environmental protection effort through riding public transportation by not polluting with one more car on the highway. If you ride an elevator, get off two flights before your floor and take the stairs. Always use the stairs over the elevator, whenever possible. If you are in good condition, trot up the stairs rather than walking.

On your lunch break, take a brisk walk around the block before you've eaten, and a leisurely one afterwards. You'll feel more alert for the rest of the day. At your desk, try to avoid sitting for too long. If you have materials that are used often and are now conveniently within reach, move them to another part of the office so that you will have to get up and fetch them. You might even consider moving your telephone across the room, or at least to a place on your desk where you will have to stand up to answer it. Don't send your secretary on your errands, do them yourself. After all, you're really not reading this book to improve your secretary's physical fitness—you want to improve your own! Use your coffee breaks to do your errands, while clearing your mind for new assignments when you get back to your desk, rather than encouraging a caffeine dependency.

Few people realize how very beneficial walking is to the body, and just as many try to avoid it at all costs. Being chauffered around from door to door may be a symbol of prestige, but time will tell when your prestige is getting the best of you. Walking gets the circulation going, breathing is improved, and it is invigorating to a tired or weary mind. Try to make it a point to take a walk every day. An ideal time for this is before dinner. If you eat dinner early (which is a good health practice), take an additional walk later in the evening, rather than collapsing on the sofa. Even your spouse can enjoy a private walk with you, not to mention how happy it will make your dog.

In later sections of the Total Glow program, specific suggestions for making exercise a part of your daily life will be presented, and some specific postures and movements will be illustrated.

Meditation: How to Do It

The technique of meditation has been around for centuries. Pinpointing the actual chronological development of the practice has been most difficult, but scholars are now placing its theoretical beginnings in the East. It spread throughout the continent of Asia, and is practiced today by people the entire world over, in one form or another.

The early Greeks and Romans were meditators, as were their future generations of philosophers and poets. Aristotle was a proponent of meditation, and often withdrew from his followers to spend extensive periods in meditative pursuits. It has been said that he absorbed himself in the practice so that he could better understand the workings of his mind through the relaxation and refreshment that it brought him.

Nearly every major religion has incorporated some form of meditation in their worship rites, although it might not be immediately recognizable as such. Some of these religions include Buddhism, Taoism, Shinto, Christianity, Judaism, and would also cover primitive religions on the American continents. In terms of the Judeo/Christian tradition, Christ meditated when he retreated into the desert for forty days. Also, the many forms of silent prayer can be placed within the major classification of meditation.

Basically, meditation is the practice of calming the mind. It is a silent, unforced guidance away from the worries and troubles of everyday life. Through it, your mind is cleared of the tension that has accumulated throughout the day, so that you are then able to start afresh.

Meditation is unstructured. A person does not actively attempt to control their thoughts or feelings while meditating. Instead, the thoughts are permitted to arise from the subconscious and, quite simply, "float away." No effort is expended in problem-solving pursuits or exercises. A thought that occurs during the process that needs a solution is merely put aside until a time when the meditator can constructively deal with it.

It is important to emphasize that meditation does not encourage repression or denial of problems or feelings; that would be antitherapeutic. Meditation is not an avoidance of problems or a method of forgetting about them. Instead it helps you to clear your mind so that you are better able to sort them out and set priorities. It also helps to reduce confusion and increase your energy level. Once meditators have calmed themselves and cleared their minds of scattered tensions and random thoughts, problem-solving becomes much easier.

Other pursuits are facilitated by meditation. What will be referred to as "spot meditation" is especially useful in the business world. In offices and organizations where stress levels are continually high due to the pressures of deadlines, interruptions, personal interactions, and performance standards, people often find the need to unwind or "regroup" before a meeting or prior to tackling an important assignment.

By simply sitting at your desk, closing your eyes, and performing a few minutes of meditation, you can effectively renew and prepare for just about anything. Obvious benefits of this would be the substantial reduction of reliance on drugs or alcohol in dealing with stress-producing situations.

Homemakers, too, can find the practice of meditation quite useful. There are many days in which the hours seem too short, or there simply aren't enough of them, when the myriad of daily tasks and responsibilities become overwhelming. When your children are napping, playing outdoors, or are at school is a perfect time to immerse yourself in meditation. It will clear your mind and renew your energy so that things don't seem quite so impossible.

Regular, daily meditation is almost doubly as beneficial as spot meditation. By freeing your mind after a busy day, you are better prepared to enjoy your leisure time in a more relaxed manner. Regular practice of meditiation also allows you to be less susceptible to tension build-up, since the stress is being released on a daily basis.

To begin meditating, there are a few initial steps which should be followed. It is important to be comfortable. Loosen tight clothing, sit in a relaxed position, try to find a spot where interruptions and noise will be minimal, and let your eyes close by themselves without forcing them shut.

The next step is to chose a "focus." In Transcendental Meditation, this is referred to as a "mantra." In keeping with the more practical Western approach, I will call it "focus"—a more explanatory word. The focus is simply a sound that you will repeat to yourself in your mind. Any word or sound will do, but it is wise to avoid ones that have connotations to you other than merely sounding pleasant. In other words, don't use the name of someone close to you, as you are not going to be concentrating on them, and don't want thoughts of them to manipulate your thoughts, or further cloud or confuse your mind.

Also, remember that the focus is not a chant. If you decide you want to use the world "money" as your focus in the hope of attracting money, you haven't quite grasped what meditation is all about. It is not a magic ritual or system of wishful or "positive" thinking at all, but merely a method of relaxation. Your focus shouldn't "mean" anything.

It should simply have a pleasant sound.

Some pleasing words without many connotations to most people might include:

celestial	sirius	estuary	terrestrial
sailing	gazelle	primrose	cumulus
aquarius	leandre	europa	irion
essence	cepheus	sheria	aurora
haven	quazar	perseus	unison
cellular	borealis	pisces	euripedes
sharing	misty	cellar	spacial

Actually, any pleasant-sounding word will suffice, and you may change, alter, or create your own focus at any time. The focus is really nothing more than a sound you will be hearing in your mind so that other random thoughts will not monopolize your meditations.

In the words of Henry Wadsworth Longfellow,

"Sit in reverie and watch the changing color of the waves that break upon the idle seashore of the mind."

This is the essence of meditation. It is the placid, peaceful, effortless observation of your mind at work releasing scurrying thoughts and tensions, and being able to enjoy the process in the bargain.

Valuable personal insight can also be gained through meditation. In effect, to watch the ways in which your mind works can offer immensely beneficial introspection. As you observe your mind ridding itself of the tensions and worries of each day, you will be able to see those areas that are particularly troublesome to you, so that you may be able to take steps to improve associations in those areas.

So, to give you an initial introduction to the technique of meditation, the following is a series of preliminary steps:

1. Find a quiet place to sit where there will be few interruptions.
2. Loosen tight clothing, remove your shoes if you wish, or simply wear a comfortable robe or kaftan.
3. Sit in a comfortable, relaxed position, but try not to slouch or place stress on any part of your body. Arms should be relaxed in your lap, resting on your legs, or on the arms of your chair.
4. Let your eyes close. Take two or three deep breaths and exhale slowly. Beginning with your feet, gradually relax each muscle in your body. Let your head bend gently forward, if that is comfortable. Relax your toes, your feet, ankles, calves, knee, thighs, buttocks, stomach, the small of your back, your chest, your shoulders, your arms, hands, fingers, neck, facial mucles,

and scalp.
5. Begin to hear your focus and let it repeat itself in your mind.

While meditating, other thoughts will crowd into your mind, but simply let them go and gradually return to your focus. This is meditation in its simplest form. It may be continued for as long as you wish, but generally, twenty minutes is the length of time most people need in order to feel relaxed and totally refreshed.

When you are finished meditating, slowly bring your mind around so that you are aware of external sensations. Open your eyes gradually, and slowly stretch and yawn. Drop your head to one side and roll it around to the other in a slow, smooth, continuous motion. Stand up and stretch again. Now you're ready to tackle anything!

Continued guidance and other relaxation enhancers will be provided throughout the book. If you did not feel as if you were meditating this first time, you can count yourself among the many thousands of first-time meditators who felt the same. Meditation is an art that takes practice, and, like most things of value, results are not instantaneous. With patience, you will find that meditation will come easier, and many experienced meditators report that they can slip into meditation on a moment's notice, whenever and wherever they choose.

At the same time, do not expect anything unusual or bizarre to happen during or after meditation. Its benefits are cumulative and you will probably find that you are feeling like a different person one day soon without having been conscious of it. You will suddenly be more relaxed, confident, capable, and better able to deal with tension and stress. This is the point at which most meditators become life-long advocates of the technique. It is called the "transition" and all who practice meditation regularly will arrive at this point sooner or later. It occurs when the cumulative benefits are recognized and it is a very enjoyable experience for most people.

Again, more information will be presented in Day #2, and you will have several more opportunities to practice. Of course, if you *did* experience a meditative state, congratulations! You are now well on the road to Total Glow and a new way of life.

Nutrition: Suggestions for Improvement

Perhaps there is nothing more confusing or controversial in today's fast-paced and rapidly changing society than the subject of food, diet, and nutrition. No sooner does one scientific study reach media attention than another one, totally refuting the first, appears and gains acceptance.

Personalities have arisen and have been replaced, while others seem to maintain their credibility. Diets like the Air Force Diet, Dr. Stillman's Diet, The Drinking Man's Diet, macrobiotics, high protein, low calorie, grapefruit, liquid protein, and water diets have come and gone. Some still have adherents.

Names like Adele Davis, Linnus Pauling, and Carlton Fredericks are no less controversial, and have attracted just as much attention from the media. The issues of Laetrile, fluoridation, and megavitamin therapy are only three areas in which public attention has been concentrated in the past decade. All of this adds up to a major public outcry for more research and much better answers.

The confusion and controversy is understandable and the public is to be congratulated for demanding more information. Also laudible is their desire to take the responsibility for their own diets. As is the case with exercise, it is only recently that people have felt the need to know more about what they are putting into their mouths.

In an agricultural society, people knew exactly what they were eating. In most cases, they could look out the window and see the hens that provided the eggs, the cows that supplied milk, and the livestock that later became their beef and pork. Even the fruit trees and vegetable crops were in plain sight. These foods were processed by hand in their own kitchens, and whatever the sanitary conditions were, or what additives went into the food, the people had direct control of it. It was never a question of peering into the contents of an aluminum can and wondering what was in it!

Today, it's a completely different story. The public is compelled to shop for food in stores where they cannot be certain of the sanitary and processing conditions. Until very recently, canned and frozen foods contained not a hint of their nutritional value. It was simply a matter of the public putting their trust in the manufacturers, canneries, and processors, assuming that they knew what they were doing. It was never even hinted that these giants might be poisoning us.

Current research is showing that poisons are indeed seeping into our bodies through commercially prepared and packaged food. Even the water supply is threatened by chemicals added for "purification" purposes. Where is all this leading, when will it stop, and what can be done about it in the meantime?

Fortunately, there are some positive answers to these questions, and you can do a great deal toward eliminating these dangerous additives and chemicals. By improving your own diet, you will be helping to clean up the entire food preparation industry. The steps are simple, and sure to bring results if enough people follow them. Until food manufacturers and processors are obliged to change their methods, the following steps can protect you and your family from what is, in reality, cumulative poisoning.

1. Read every label before you buy a product. Know what you are eating and feeding your family. Do some research into those additives which have been proved harmful, and refuse to buy foods containing them.
2. Refuse to buy foodstuffs that are essentially lacking in nutritional value. This group would consist mainly of commercial snacks, packaged/processed/frozen convenience foods, and the many breads, flours, and cereals that are almost wholly comprised of bleached flour, chemicals, salt, and sugar.
3. Refuse to patronize (or patronize less often) those companies, stores, and restaurants that offer only highly-processed junk foods.
4. Adapt the attitude that you will work toward changing your eating habits through sensible healthful foods, and learn how to prepare delicious, nutritious meals for yourself that are not only easy, but are time-saving as well. Attitude and responsibility are vitally important to this program.
5. Try to introduce these concepts to those people around you whom you care about, but do this gradually so they won't feel as if they are being pushed into something they may not like.

The ways in which to achieve these goals are clearly outlined in the Total Glow program, and continuing information will be provided throughout the book. At this time, however, it is interesting to take a look at the ways our culture views food and "diet."

It is a widespread misconception that the word "diet" refers only to something a person does who is desireous of losing weight. Usually the word brings to mind endless days of plain tea, dry toast, and cottage cheese. It has become associated with deprivation through common usage, but actually the word refers to *anything that is consumed regularly.*

Therefore, the phrase "national diet" does not mean a weight-loss program in which the entire country is participating, but rather to the types of food the country normally consumes. The diet of the United States is heavily concentrated on the protein and carbohydrates found in red meat, breads, and processed cereals. In addition, we consume more soft drinks and fast foods than any other culture. Conversely, the

Asian diet consists to a greater degree than ours of fish and vegetables. (Interestingly, Asian women have far less breast cancer than American women, but when they move to the U.S., their rate greatly increases.)

To have each person realize this and take the responsibility for their own individual diet is the goal of this program. When you can accept the fact that you alone are responsible for the food that you eat, you will be better able to make beneficial changes in your health. It is helpful to remember that perhaps the only people in this country who have no control over their diets are children, and those in institutions where they must eat what is served, or go without.

An Historical Look at Food

In most cultures of the world, there is a tremendous amount of importance placed upon food which is above and beyond the mere consumption of it. Consider for a moment the many ways in which we celebrate happy occasions or good fortune. Many of us will go-out-to-dinner to celebrate an anniversary, birthday, or some other happy occasion. It would probably be impossible to count the number of vitally important business transactions that have been concluded over a meal; ranging from the typical business lunch to grand affairs at the White House.

Most of this country's religious and national holidays are centered around a feast of some sort. At Christmastime there is usually a gigantic meal with a turkey, stuffing, potatoes, breads, pies, cookies, candies, and such beverages as egg nog. Thanksgiving carries with it a similar bill of fare. On the Fourth of July, the large family picnic is traditional, with hot dogs, hamburgers, potato and macaroni salads, potato chips, corn on the cob, strawberry shortcake, and other desserts. During Easter celebrations, many families observe the holiday with a meal consisting of ham, sweet potatoes with marshmallow topping—and this isn't even to mention the chocolate eggs and jelly beans! During the Jewish observation of Passover, the typical menu consists of motza, eggs, gefelte fish, chicken soup with motza balls, chicken, and honey cake.

It's easy to see that by making taste buds feel good and stomachs full, this country celebrates happy occasions.

A Psychological Look at Food

It is worth consideration, too, as an indication of the ways in which our society is food- and sweet-oriented, the terms of endearment we have for each other. People are taught (however subconsciously) from their earliest days that something sweet is "good." This applies to moral issues as well. When speaking to loved ones, the terms *sweetheart, honey, sugar, sweetie,* and other "sugary" terms are used. Imagine how hard this orientation is to overcome by a person trying to control their weight, when they believe almost instrinsically that all sweet things and all feasts mean that they are good people and that they are loved. How many times have you seen an adult give a child candy for being "good"?

It is not my intention to try to change your way of thinking about holidays and love-terms. If these times and things are enjoyable to you, great! I hope that each person can accomplish recognition of their greatest potential and best state of health through consciously being aware of what they eat. Often, it is advantageous to point out the pitfalls along the way, especially when they concern deep psychological biases.

Since many aspects of food and nutrition are unknown or vastly misunderstood by many people, it is my intent to provide you with the results of many years of research, trial and error, and successes. Most of all, I want you to discover that taking care of your body and overall health can be one of the most enjoyable and satisfying endeavors you have ever experienced.

The following questions are designed to help you become more aware of your general state of health, your feelings, and your knowledge in this area.

As you go through the questions, really think about each one. Take a few minutes to formulate your answer to each of them. This way, you will gain a tremendous amount of knowledge about yourself and the ways in which you are currently thinking and reacting to the world around you.

Too many people are so used to feeling bad that they have forgotten what it feels like to be in good health, both physically and emotionally. Basically, we are anesthetized and cut off from our feelings. We are taught that aging brings all the ailments we feel are a natural part of getting old. If we are so willing to accept this teaching, I wonder why some of us aren't as willing to accept the idea that eating natural food is a natural process of life as well. We *can* take care of ourselves and make our lives infinitely better!

The Total Glow Health Questionnaire
A Self Test
To Determine Your Physical And Emotional Health

	Yes	No
1. Are you a positive person? Do you look forward to each day when you awaken?	☐	☐
2. Do you feel relaxed and in a positive frame of mind, even after putting in a full day's work?	☐	☐
3. Do you spend your time constructively, but in a way that is enjoyable to you?	☐	☐
4. Can you show love, admiration, or goodwill for other people easily?	☐	☐
5. Do you feel joyous very often?	☐	☐
6. Do you look and feel healthy?	☐	☐
7. Are you able to handle your emotions in unpleasant situations?	☐	☐
8. Do you look forward to the future?	☐	☐
9. Are you tolerant of other people?	☐	☐
10. Do you enjoy sex?	☐	☐
11. Do you enjoy physical contact?	☐	☐
12. Can you make everyday decisions easily?	☐	☐
13. Are you honest in your dealings with people on all levels—social, business, and family?	☐	☐
14. Do you seek out interesting people from whom you can learn about new and different things?	☐	☐
15. Do you usually feel full of energy?	☐	☐
16. Do you often feel a vague but omnipresent sense of guilt?	☐	☐
17. Do you blame yourself for things beyond your control or blame others for your own failings?	☐	☐

18. If you were someone else, how would that person describe you? _____

_____

19. How do you take criticism? _____

_____

20. Are you able to laugh and smile often? Do you have a good sense of humor?	☐	☐

	Yes	No

21. Are you more than five pounds overweight? ☐ ☐
22. Are there any specific habits you would like to break? ☐ ☐
23. Do you ever have trouble falling asleep or sleeping through the night? ☐ ☐
24. Have you noticed a few bumps and bulges that were never there before? ☐ ☐
25. Do you seem to have less energy than you once had? ☐ ☐
26. Do you ever feel anxious, irritable, or edgy for no apparent reason? ☐ ☐
27. Do you know how much refined sugar you ingest on an average day? ☐ ☐
28. Do you know how much salt you ingest on an average day? ☐ ☐
29. Do you know the dangers of overconsumption of sugar and salt? ☐ ☐
30. Do you ever have trouble saying "no" to requests made of you, when you don't want to fulfill those requests? ☐ ☐
31. Is the potato a food to be avoided when you are trying to lose weight? ☐ ☐
32. Is walking a good way to lose weight? ☐ ☐
33. Is commercial yogurt good for you? ☐ ☐
34. Do the kinds of clothes you wear jogging make much difference? ☐ ☐
35. Are wheat germ and wheat germ oil good for you? ☐ ☐
36. Do you have to get your heart beating rapidly and work up a sweat for exercise to be any good at all? ☐ ☐

Answers and Discussion

Although there are no strict "right" or "wrong" answers to many of the above questions, they are here primarily to give you an overall picture of yourself and the areas where you may feel the need to improve. Many times people will not really recognize a problem until they take an evaluation test like the one above. If you answered some of the questions in a way that indicates a need for improvement, check them over to see exactly where these areas might be. Are they mainly physical, social/emotional, or a combination of both?

Below is a discussion of each of the questions, and an explanation of the ways in which the Total Glow program can help you.

1. *Are you a positive person? Do you look forward to each day when you awaken?*

Very few of us bound out of bed each morning full of energy and enthusiasm, and you needn't expect to do the same. However, if one or two times a week you wake up unrested or feeling as if each day is just another twenty-four hours to suffer through, then emotionally and/or physically, your health is below par.

2. *Do you feel relaxed and in a positive frame of mind, even after putting in a full day's work?*

Most people begin to drag at about six o'clock in the evening and come home feeling frazzled and irritable. But just because most people feel this way does not mean that it is normal. It may be average for our population, but in a country of unhealthy people, average is not necessarily normal. Ten to twenty minutes of exercise and/or self-relaxation as recommended in the Total Glow program will help you renew your energy.

3. *Do you spend your time constructively and in a way that is enjoyable to you?*

"Workaholics" are those who feel compelled to toil away at something every waking hour in order to allay the guilt they will feel if they do "nothing." Often they don't really enjoy their projects and labors as much as they could, but cannot reconcile the "waste" of time they would spend watching television, reading, or simply steeped in thought. Others tend to spend their free time vegetating on the sofa with little or no ambition to lift a finger. If you have trouble reconciling work and play, it is time you took a closer look at what you are doing to yourself physically and emotionally, and how it may be effecting those around you.

4. *Can you show love, admiration, or goodwill for other people easily?*

For any number of reasons, tense people are usually afraid to express their feelings of friendship, affection, and goodwill. Men, particularly, sometimes feel as if displays of emotion are not masculine. This leads to more isolation, loneliness, and lack of trust. People will soon stop expressing positive feelings to you. You may wonder why "no one likes you" or includes you in activities any longer.

5. *Do you feel joyous very often?*

In the same way that tense people put a damper on their feelings toward other people, they also stifle their own emotions such as exhiliration, joy, and anticipation. On the other hand, they turn their backs on sorrow and grief as well. In effect, they are not feeling anything. These people walk around in a state of numbness and do not allow themselves to deviate to either extreme. To feel the pinnacle of joy, one must also know what it is like to experience great sorrow. The Total Glow program encourages you to open up and experience the deeper levels of emotion. As you do this, you will find that nothing "bad" happens if you allow yourself to feel.

6. *Do you look and feel healthy?*

If your physique isn't really in the best shape it could be, you are showing signs of premature aging, or your face has lost its healthy shine, chances are that you've let your self-esteem slip as well. It is time that you checked yourself to see what precipitated this, otherwise your health will continue to deteriorate.

7. *Are you able to handle your emotions in unpleasant situations?*

Grief, anger, and joy are appropriate emotions in appropriate situations, but do you find that your anger sometimes explodes at people or things that are not the cause of it? Do you find yourself sobbing over a sad movie when problems closer to home go ignored? Many times, the denial of the existence of these strong emotions leads to the inappropriate expression of them (i.e. the sad movie). People often make the assumption that simply because they allow themselves to feel angry, they will perform an "angry" act, which really isn't so. Observe yourself next time you are sad or angry, and see if you are reacting appropriately.

8. *Do you look forward to the future?*

When we are so deeply ensnared in anxiety about the past and present, we cannot possibly afford the time to contemplate the future. Most people spend their lives regretting yesterday and worrying about tomorrow, or living for tomorrow and not enjoying today. The old phrase, "When I finish," is their trap. When the kids are in school, when the kids are grown up and gone, when I retire—these phrases have trapped them and they will soon find that life has passed them by. Start looking into what extent your life is wasted in this manner and begin to change it.

9. *Are you tolerant of other people?*

No one expects you to embrace everyone you meet with open arms like a long-lost friend, but maintaining an open mind about acquaintances, co-workers, and relatives is the outcome of a healthy, relaxed state of mind. Also, being open and relaxed enough, and secure in yourself to the extent that you are tolerant of other people's value and styles is the outcome of health.

10. *Do you enjoy sex?*

Sexual dysfunctions are often caused by tension and stress that have too long been allowed free reign, or anxieties that have been suppressed. Buried feelings of anger or guilt can also cause sexual problems, where we are not able to experience full sexual pleasure. Many who are physically out of shape feel embarrassment and lack of energy. As a more relaxed and physically fit person, you can experience yourself and your partner more fully.

11. *Do you enjoy physical contact?*

While no one enjoys strangers or casual acquaintances constantly putting their hands on them, the need for physical contact is as old as the human race. Gentle touching is a way of showing affection and closeness, especially in appreciation. When you know someone and care about them, touching them is a way of telling them your feelings. Remember that human infants can waste away and die if they are not touched and cradled by another human being. And almost all of us can remember how good it felt to be hugged by Mom or Dad when we were frightened or skinned our knees.

12. *Can you make everyday decisions easily?*

Whether or not to cash in your savings bonds for the downpayment on a house is not an everyday decision, but deciding what to order for lunch or what movie to see is one. Any type of decision often throws some of us into a quandary, because of the fear of making the wrong choice. These people most often prefer to let others make their decisions for them, which points out a lack of self-esteem. It's also important to remember that you always have the right to change your mind.

13. *Are you honest in your dealings with people on all levels—social, business, and family?*

Being brutally frank and harsh with your employees and co-workers while walking on eggs with your spouse is really no way to get along with yourself as a totally integrated person. Neither is gritting your teeth and suffering insults from your in-laws in silence, when you are usually assertive and fair with most other people. Observe your dealings with people on all levels.

14. *Do you seek out interesting people from whom you can learn about new and different things?*

The wallflower syndrome is a typical outcome of an uptight person. At the same time, people who intentionally close their minds to new ideas and experiences are too tense to accept any change in their unnecessarily hectic minds. Also, lack of energy and vitality can result in boredom, which is a killer.[1] Try to open yourself up to new ideas, and avoid making snap judgements about things until you know more about them.

15. *Do you usually feel full of energy?*

If you usually get enough sleep and are eating properly, you ought to be feeling fine most of the time. If you feel as if you are on the verge of exhaustion more than once or twice a week, it is probably due to excess nervous tension, improper diet, or that your system is overloading with unnecessary toxins which your body is trying to fight off. By following the suggestions in the Total Glow program, you can develop your mind and rid your body of poisons so that they can work together in a calm, efficient manner.

16. *Do you often feel a vague but omnipresent sense of guilt?*

Guilt is a destructive, *learned* aspect of the human condition. It is when guilt is experienced for no real reason and when it becomes overpowering that depression sets in and we find ourselves in trouble. The Total Glow program can give you plenty to feel GOOD about, so that you will be better able to deal realistically with guilt feelings. In

---

[1]Valid and continued research tends to indicate that personality traits may play an important part in cancer development. Studies by researchers such as Dr. L. Le Shan of the Institute of Applied Biology at New York University, Dr. Arthur Schmale, Jr., Dr. Howard Iker, and Dr. Greene of the University of Rochester Medical Center, all came up with similar findings; certain types of people, those with a lowered ability to handle stress and severe emotional conflicts, people with uncontrolled anxieties and worries, with traumatic emotional experiences or losses, are more prone to disease. People suffering from loneliness, hopelessness, boredom (which underneath is a lack of self-esteem or, in other words, inadequacy and helplessness), are more likely than others to develop diseases, including cancer. Although such a negative mind state may not in itself cause cancer, the increase in hopelessness and the desire for what I call a "zest for life" may lead to susceptibility and increased biochemical vulnerability that lowers the body's resistance and therefore helps set the stage for the growth of cancer.

Lawrence Le Shan, *Cancer and Personality: A Critical Review* (Journal of the National Cancer Institute, 1959), and Howard R. Lewis and Martha E. Lewis, *Psychosomatics* (New York: Viking Press, Inc.)

addition to this, it should be emphasized that this program can help clear your mind so that you are not so susceptible to accepting unwarranted guilt. Some people will place guilt on another, and that person will (consciously or unconsciously) accept it. Try to become more aware of what is happening, so that you will not feel the need to repress guilt feelings and can therefore *really* help yourself.

17. *Do you usually blame yourself for things beyond your control, or blame others for your failings?*

Although these two behavioral patterns may seem diametrically opposed to each other, they are closely related in a psychological sense. Accepting undue blame or "passing the buck" can be equally destructive in certain circumstances. If you are either continually apologizing for things that are not your fault, or blaming your failings on someone else, you are holding an unrealistic view of yourself and others. Constant apologizing is also a cry for attention, and can become quite annoying to other people, finally producing the opposite effect. You need to take time to watch and explore your behavior and differentiate between those things you are actually responsible for, and those that you are not.

18. *If you were someone else, how would that person describe you?*

In psychology, the term "Looking Glass Self" describes a subconscious method whereby people get to know themselves through the reactions and feedback from people with whom they come in contact. We come to know what we are like by the "reflections" seen of ourselves in other people. Tense and nervous people often cannot read themselves in others' reactions or body language because they block out these messages. Their minds are racing too fast in non-constructive pursuits and are too cluttered to pick up these subliminal reflections. Try to listen and pay attention to other people's reactions to you.

19. *How do you take criticism?*

Have you ever caught yourself flying into a rage or dissolving into tears when someone criticizes you or your work? Are you over-sensitive to criticism? Confidence and the building of self-esteem are integral parts of the Total Glow program, whereby criticism becomes easier to deal with effectively.

20. *Are you able to laugh and smile often? Do you have a good sense of humor?*

Laughter is the greatest tension reliever known to the human race. It is no mistake that most speakers or lecturers open with a joke just to get the audience relaxed. Laughter is, in fact, unique among humans. Through it, people obtain a release; they are able to laugh at themselves easily and see the humor in many situations. Of course, walking around with a silly grin on your face will be likely to arouse suspicion as to your mental faculties, but an appropriate smile shows that you are relaxed and that you are listening. It also makes an astounding difference in personal interactions when a smile is added to the conversation. As your body becomes healthier inside and out through following the Total Glow program, you will present a friendlier, happier, more relaxed appearance to the world because it will reflect your inner health and contentment.

21. *Are you more than five pounds overweight?*

Physical appearance is almost always an indicator of our feelings of self-esteem. An unattractive appearance, whether it be an overweight or unkempt one, tells the world that you don't care much about yourself. Being underweight can also be saying that you don't care enough to eat properly or that you are ill. Either way, this program can help you achieve and maintain a glowing, healthy body that bespeaks of your inherent sense of self-worth.

22. *Are there any specific habits you would like to break?*

You know what your bad habits are, and chances are that you've tried to break them in the past. Most often, destructive habits (such as smoking, overeating, overindulging in drink or drugs) are the outcome of nervous or anxious states of mind. Using self-relaxation, try to calm yourself to the point where you can analyze your habits and take constructive steps toward becoming free of them.

23. *Do you ever have trouble falling asleep or sleeping through the night?*

Insomnia afflicts thousands of people and the "cures" are filling up the druggist's shelves. Although we generally need less sleep as we grow older, there are still enough of us who feel the need for drugs in order to get a full night's rest. Sleep difficulties are most often the symptoms of unresolved conflicts and/or poor eating habits. Improper sugar metabolism frequently causes people to awaken too early. The Total Glow program can aid you in eliminating the worry these conflicts cause and also, when you are more active and healthy, sleep is never difficult.

24. *Have you noticed a few bumps and bulges that were never there before?*

Now is the time to start doing something about them! As we mature, our bodies require less and less food, yet most of us simply continue eating the same amount of food we ate as teenagers. The exercises and directions for healthful eating in this program will enable you to get a head start on weight and figure problems before they become serious.

25. *Do you seem to have less energy than you did before?*

When your body is out of condition, when you are carrying around excess poundage, and when the most exercise you've given yourself in the past month was to ride up an elevator, no wonder you don't have any energy! Trim down, shape up, get moving, detoxify your body—these are the goals of the Total Glow program, and I will show you how to go about achieving them.

26. *Do you ever feel anxious, irritable, or edgy for no apparent reason?*

Unless you are faced with an immediate, concrete, stressful situation, it is not normal to feel anxious. General nervousness or anxiety is quite often caused by improper eating habits or through an unsettled, tense state of mind. When you notice periods of anxiety, irritability, or edginess, try to correlate them with something you've eaten (or not eaten), or with some other general worry that is bothering you.

27. *Do you know how much refined sugar you ingest on an average day?*

Even if you were to eliminate all sweets and sugar from your diet entirely, you would still be ingesting more than you think. So much refined sugar is disguised in chemical language that the average person cannot and does not understand exactly how much refined sugar he/she is putting into their bodies. Refined sugar has been the villain in many physical and emotional disorders, as you will discover as you go through the Total Glow program. The average consumption of sugar in the U.S. is 110 pounds per person per year.

28. *Do you know how much salt you ingest on an average day?*

As with sugar (though salt is not disguised as much), you are probably getting a great deal more than you think. Salt is put into processed foods to make them taste better, because most of the original flavor has been cooked out. The Total Glow program has some suggestions along the lines of reducing your salt intake. The average consumption is nine to ten grams per day per person. Our essential requirement is one half gram.

29. *Do you know the dangers of overconsumption of sugar and salt?*

As mentioned earlier, refined sugar is an addictive, harmful substance that can cause irreputable harm. In fact, you could live longer on a diet of water only, than on one of water and refined sugar. Most of us know the problems caused by too much salt; water retention, high blood pressure, and heart disease included. The Total Glow program helps you re-evaluate your use of these two substances and provides guidelines for kicking the habits.

30. *Do you ever have trouble saying "no" to requests made of you when you do not want to fulfill those requests?*

The ability to say "no" pleasantly and tactfully when someone asks you to do something you don't want to do is the essence of assertiveness. But before effective assertion is possible, a sense of self-esteem must be realized. The building of self-esteem and feelings of self-worth is an integral part of this program.

31. *Is the potato a food to be avoided when you are trying to lose weight?*

Surprisingly, the potato is a good all-around food. Actually it is only when we French fry it, make chips out of it, or hash brown it that the potato becomes less healthful. The composition of a potato is 0.1% fat, lots of vitamin C, many elements of the B-complex, and other minerals, proteins, and fiber. As for protein, its quality equals that of wheat; a medium potato contains 20% of our R.D.A. Furthermore, studies relating to consumption of this vegetable show that not one subject has shown an increase in weight, even when potatoes were the only food consumed for up to ten weeks. Since Americans eat more potatoes than oranges (which are one of the best sources of Vitamin C), the potato is a major source of Vitamin C in this country. Always eat them with the skins, for the vitamins and minerals are concentrated there. Potato chips have lost 75% of their nutrients, mashed potatoes in frozen dinners have lost 80%, and baked or boiled potatoes have lost only 22% and 19% respectively.[2]

32. *Is walking a good way to lose weight?*

Walking is an excellent way to lose weight gradually, although it burns up relatively few calories. The heavier you are, the more calories you will burn, and men use up more than women. If you figure that about 150 calories are burned per half hour of walking, you will experience a weight loss of fifteen to twenty pounds in a year's time of walking an hour per day, *with no change in food intake*. You will also be toning your muscles and helping your respiratory and circulatory systems immeasurably. You can see, then, how a walking schedule could be much more beneficial than a year's worth of crash diets.

33. *Is commercial yogurt good for you?*

The key word here is "commercial." Most of these yogurts do not contain the bacteria lactobacillus acidophillus. In experiments with laboratory animals, lactobacillus acidophillus has been shown to reduce the levels of three floral enzymes involved in the formation of cancer-causing substances in the intestinal tract. Thus, yogurt con-

---

[2]*Prevention*, "The Greasing of the Spud." May, 1978.

taining lactobacillus acidophillus is believed to help prevent cancer of the colon and large bowel. Without this bacteria, commercial yogurt cannot be as beneficial as natural yogurts. Also, most commercial yogurts are heavily sweetened with processed fruits and refined sugar.

34. Do the kinds of clothes you wear jogging make much difference?

Jogging clothes, as with any sport, are very important, though they need not be expensive. Usually cotton shorts and cotton tee shirts are best in warm weather. In colder climates, wear loose-fitting warm up suits and try to avoid sweat pants or other baggy attire that will get in your way and could trip you. I recommend that women wear good, well-fitting bras, as the stress placed upon the soft tissues of the breast while jogging could cause them to tear. Jogging shoes are of utmost importance. The shoes will be the biggest investment you will need to make, and can usually be found for less than $40. Shoes especially made for jogging can save you from foot, ankle, shin, and knee injuries.

35. Are wheat germ and wheat germ oils good for you?

They are healthy, but the thing to bear in mind is that wheat germ, wheat germ oil, and whole wheat flour are subject to rancidity more rapidly than most foods. Rancid foods may be a cause of cancer. If you can be certain that wheat germ products are no fewer than four days old, they are indeed very healthy and good for you.

36. Do you have to get your heart beating rapidly and work up a sweat before exercise is any good at all?

No, not in the beginning. Strenuous exercise will do you more harm than good at this point. As mentioned earlier, walking is great exercise and I recommend it to everyone, young and old alike. The exercises presented in the Total Glow program are ones that will tone your body quickly without alot of muscle aches and soreness. Once you are in better physical condition, you will probably feel like performing more strenuous exercises, including aerobics.

Everyone wants to be healthier, happier, and better able to deal with the tensions of the world in which we live. The Total Glow program can make a big difference in your life. Its goal, as outlined in this book, will enable you to develop into a totally integrated, healthy person with a greater sense of self-esteem.

Any further, more specific goals that you might have may also be incorporated into the program. Included in this book are progress-checking methods, space to record your experiences with the program, and self-testing methods through which you can determine your knowledge and awareness.

By helping you learn to relax, a lessened desire to over-indulge in food, drink, and drugs will gradually become apparent to you. As you rid your body of chemical toxins and begin to tone your muscles, a feeling of better health and vitality will prevail. All of these aspects are important and inter-related. They work in conjunction to produce a healthier, happier you.

Any self-improvement plan, however, depends mainly upon those individuals who attempt it. It may be adapted to be a quick, intense process through which you can gain timely results, or the choice might be made to make this program a part of your everyday life from this point forward. The latter option is suggested, since the benefits received from this program are ones that will greatly enhance life in terms of your zest for living, self-esteem, health, and in your dealings with other people.

Now that you have finished the first day and this health questionnaire, I suggest that you take a closer look at yourself. List some of your specific goals. Think of five things you can do tomorrow that have already been suggested. List them and plan to do at least three.

Day 2
The Plan

The Importance of Relaxation—How Your Personality Affects Your Health

Meditation as a form of relaxation, has been included in the Total Glow program because I find it to be an effective relaxation technique that can be learned and practiced by the greatest number of people, at the lowest cost.

The type of meditation outlined in this book enables you to reach a greater level of relaxation than would otherwise be experienced during rest or sleep. This form of meditation allows you to function more efficiently, creatively, and, therefore, happily, in all facets of life through regular practice.

Meditation is a *portable* relaxation technique in that it can go with you anywhere, in whatever method or variation you choose to adopt. It can be tailored so that you can benefit from it however and whenever you so desire, and most people have found that regular practice of the technique increases their enjoyment of life, their health, and their productivity.

Since meditation is one of the best ways of reducing stress, many physicians believe that it can be an aid in treating psychosomatic illnesses. Heart disease, reactive high blood pressure, arthritis, the many varieties of muscular tension (migraine, low back pain, and gastrointestinal disorders), and asthma, can be the direct result of accumulated stress, or can be gravely complicated by anxiety. It has been theorized that even some forms of cancer might be brought on or accelerated by anxious states of mind.[1]

If you were to observe the people around you closely, you would probably come to the conclusion that those who are ill most frequently

---

[1]Lawrence Le Shan, *Cancer and Personality: A Critical Review,* Op. Cit.

with minor complaints are those who tend to be the most nervous or worried. It has been theorized as well that common, everyday illnesses such as colds and flu might be precipitated by tension because the body's combative abilities are diminished. There are always exceptions to this rule, however. If a person never *admits* that he/she is sick or in pain, or does not allow him- or herself the knowledge of his/her illness, that is a different story. But this phenomenon, too, can be attributed to high-level stress.

Certainly, there is a great need for the public to find an outlet for their accumulated anxieties.

For a great number of people, meditation is the answer. Let me share with you the experiences of a few of the subjects who have already followed the meditation plan which I outline in this book. The following is a short case history of one person who had a particular stress situation and found that meditation was an aid in overcoming it.

Case History I: Benefits of Spot Meditation

"I had always found it difficult to travel by car for even short distances. While attending college (which was an eight-hour drive on interstate highways, back when everybody was going 70 miles per hour), I saw so many accidents that I just couldn't relax while I was in a car.

"It got so bad that I wouldn't even consider visiting friends or relatives if it meant going by car on the interstate. I really couldn't imagine anything worse than spending hours in a car.

"The situation got worse when we moved to this area and had to get to work on the interstate. I started back-seat driving and was a wreck by the time I finally got to work or got home.

"When I heard about meditation and Dr. Rona's program, I wondered if I could use the technique to help myself get over my fear of car travel. Dr. Rona suggested that I try it, and I did. On a recent trip to see relatives, I felt the same old tenseness coming on. So I lowered the seat in the car, closed my eyes, and started relaxing with the meditation technique.

"Needless to say, I was relaxed throughout the whole trip, and was able to enjoy myself much more when we arrived."

This is but one example of the multitude of benefits of meditation, and the flexibility with which it may be utilized. There may be similar situations in your life where you may use it to overcome a fear or stress-producing situation. The regular practice of meditation, as opposed to this example of spot meditation, will most likely reduce your anxiety about most situations and activities, making you a more relaxed person overall.

Another story of the myriad of benefits comes from a businessman in his middle forties:

Case History II: One Businessman's Story

"Frankly, for the past twenty years, I've had so little time to myself that if somebody told me to relax, I wouldn't have known what they were talking about. When I used to go on vacation with my family, I thought about nothing but my work and getting ahead. I certainly enjoyed my career (I always have), but I was paying a price.

"I was smoking two packs of cigarettes a day, I had high blood pressure, headaches, irritability, and poor concentration. Too many things were building up. What bothered me most was that I was growing old. Fast. I wasn't paying enough attention to my family either. If they did get attention, I was usually barking at them for one thing or another. It's a wonder they didn't desert me.

"Anyway, I'm so skeptical, I didn't trust anybody or their solutions, especially the ones that seemed to be way out. All that talk about meditation seemed like another passing fad for the kids.

"But I guess I was wrong. My kids eventually let me know in their own way that I was missing out on life's real pleasures. They talked about meditation and brought home a couple of books about it. I softened up and started to read a few.

"Then I heard about Dr. Rona's more practical approach and decided to give it a try. I realized that I could tailor it to my way of life, and didn't have to subscribe to alot of foreign religious ideals.

"At first, I felt like an A-One fool sitting there all by myself saying this word over and over in my head. But after a while I changed my tune. My days seemed longer and fuller and I started noticing alot of changes. Little things don't bother me as much and I started to have more energy. I cut down on my smoking and social drinking, mainly because I was so relaxed that I really didn't need it as much.

"What I think I appreciate most is that for the first time in years, my health is in a much better state than it's been in a long time. If a few minutes of total relaxation can work for somebody like me, I'm sure it can work pretty much for everybody."

In recent years, women have gained greater access to advancement opportunities in the business world. They are continually seeking greater and greater authority and positions of power. The number of women moving up from the ranks of secretaries and clerical workers is growing rapidly.

With this advancement, however, comes the stress that male businesspeople have had to cope with for years. Few women have been taught the ways in which to handle this "executive stress" syndrome, and this is where meditation can be a tangible asset to aspiring women.

This is how one recently promoted executive put it:

Case History III: A Young Executive's Experience

"I found I was working harder and harder and going home worn to a frazzle. I didn't have time to be interested in anything else, because I was so exhausted all the time. When I did try to get back to my hobbies, I caught myself trying to rush through them—which wasn't relaxing or enjoyable at all!

"At work I was fine—calm, competent, hard-working—but my homelife was in shambles. When I discovered meditation, I was very skeptical at first. A friend told me about her experiences with TM, but I was still too turned off by the impracticality of it. Then I heard about Dr. Rona's form of meditation, and decided that I'd give it a try.

"Let me tell you that I must have been the toughest customer she ever had. For one thing, I didn't have time to pursue anything that wasn't going to show immediate results. After a few attempts, though, I could see that meditation was really working. I felt much better all around. I started to realize that what I thought was brilliance at work would eventually put me in an early grave.

"Now I'm more relaxed, can work better at a less frantic pace. Best of all, meditation freed my mind of all the little inconsequential things so that I feel I have more time for my hobbies and pasttimes. My husband has even noticed a big difference!

"Since I really don't have time to meditate each and every day, I'll usually sit for a few minutes at my desk before getting into my work. It's great for emptying my mind of all the little tensions and worries and preparing myself for some clear thinking.

"I really wouldn't be without meditation now, it's made such a difference in my life."

As an outcome of many years of inquiry and scientific research, a growing number of psychologists and therapists are recommending meditation to their patients who suffer from high level stress. In addition to its ability to reduce or alleviate tension, meditation produces some rather pronounced changes which further enhance the benefits of relaxation.

Some of the institutions where the physiological aspects of meditation are being studied are Harvard University, the University of California at Irvine, and Tubbingen in West Germany. Early in 1935, a French cardiologist named Therese Brosse travelled to India to investigate the yogis and their experiences with meditative states.

Equipped with a portable electrocardiograph, she found after intensive study that one particular yogi was willfully able to stop his heartbeat and then start it again on command. Other studies have come to similar, quite startling conclusions. In essence, this might reinforce the currently intriguing idea of mind over matter, especially where the body is concerned.

These types of feats are not the aim of most meditators, however, nor is this type of extreme the aim of the Total Glow program. It is mentioned simply to illustrate the ways in which the mind and body can be and are used effectively in harmony with each other.

The most significant study made on the physiological effects of meditation was performed by Rober Keith Wallace with Herbert Benson, through work supported by grants from the National Institute of Health. In their articles, "The Physiology of Meditation," published in *Scientific American Offprints,* they came to some interesting conclusions, including meditation's effect on brain wave activity. The following information is drawn from that report.

The Four Levels of Brain Wave Activity

At the present time, four levels of brain wave activity have been identified and categorized. Their structure correlates to a higher, more comprehensive system of brain evolution where each level slowly developed toward the potential for a "higher" human with greater intelligence. The levels are Beta, Alpha, Theta, and Delta.

> Beta—14 to 21 cycles per second
> Alpha—7 to 14 cycles per second
> Theta—4 to 7 cycles per second
> Delta—0 to 4 cycles per second

The most conscious and cognizant level of brain activity is the Beta level. This is the level at which your brain is operating as you read this book. It is associated with the sensations of sight, sound, smell, and taste. Cycles of brain waves, measured on an electroencelphalograph, in this state are the highest frequency and occur at a rate of between fourteen and twenty-one cycles per second. Other studies in mind activity claim that the number of cycles in the Beta level is even higher, and can range as high as forty per second.

The next slower frequency is the Alpha level. This is where meditation occurs. It is the level at which the inner consciousness is not aware of time or space, and it is associated with tranquility, rest, and deep relaxation. Alpha is also linked with the concept of memory, reflection, and dreaming. Some studies of parapsychology associate this level with extrasensory perception.

Below Alpha is the Theta level, which is presently catagorized as the subconscious state. It may be the most creative, problem-solving level of mind activity, and it is in this state to which people descend when hypnotized, or anesthetized for surgery or childbirth. It seems that great creative imagination, inspiration, and insight arise from this level and psychologists are attempting to explain the significance of the dreams that emerge from it. Studies have been conducted to determine whether or not dreams are significant problem-solving symbolisms through which the subconscious mind attempts to inform the conscious mind of ways in which to better deal with problems and worries.

(Some people have found it enlightening to record their dreams each morning upon awakening. After a month or so, it is quite interesting to read back over the dreams and attempt to recognize some kind of pattern. Although debate is still raging over Dr. Sigmund Freud's interpretation of dreams and the human being's psycho-sexual development theory, continuing research into the investigation of dreams and their interpretation can be a valuable psychotherapeutic tool, and it can help you understand yourself better throughout your entire life.)

The very deep sleep in which dreams occur with most frequency is the Theta level, which has brain wave cycles of between four and seven per second.

The next slower level is Delta, and this is believed to be the deepest part of the subconscious mind. Little research has been performed in the investigation of this level, and it is known only that it does indeed exist. Speech, thought, and any form of rational or voluntary action is non-existant in Delta. It has been found that newborn infants spend most of their time in Delta, where there are from zero to four cycles per second.

In Japan, studies performed with meditators showed a slowing of the Alpha waves from the usual frequency of seven to fourteen cycles per second to seven or eight cycles. At this point, Theta waves (at six cycles per second) appeared, showing that the subjects were in an extremely deep state of relaxation. As they emerged from meditation, their brain wave cycles returned to the Alpha level, but were calmer.

Psychological Aspects of Meditation

Other physiological changes occurring during meditation include a lowering of oxygen consumption, blood lactate level, and metabolic rate. Since all these biological processes are accelerated or complicated by stress, the effects of meditation in slowing them down is clearly beneficial. In the future, further research into meditation will undoubtedly reveal more numerous effects and benefits. The above information is only a fraction of the research data that will be gathered in coming years as meditation becomes an integral part of the lives of thousands of people.

There are a number of noticeable physical and psychological effects that have been reported to take place after beginning the practice of meditation. Some of these changes are apparent after the very first attempt, while others take longer to be recognized.

Of all the people who have practiced the form of meditation presented in the Total Glow program, each one reported an immediate, overall feeling of better health. Many said they experienced a feeling of superior muscle coordination, and several practitioners (who are over fifty years of age) reported an increased energy level and a desire to engage in more physical activity.

Because the nervous system is relaxed during meditation, one of the effects noticed by a great number of people is an improved memory. Although meditation may be on a different brain wave cycle level than dreaming, the process correlates somewhat with the way in which memories, images, words, and ideas are stored in the subconscious and subsequently brought to the surface. Mental stress blocks memory, and meditation reduces stress, giving the mind a chance to bring forth stored information.

Basic and elemental calming of the mind and nervous system through meditation can bring about many beneficial changes in your personality. One of the most noticeable is increased self-confidence. Another benefit is the ability to enjoy all aspects of life through reduction of stress and the opening up of acceptance for your life's ups and downs.

To help you in your second attempt at meditation, the basic steps to the technique will be outlined once again to re-familiarize you with it. A refinement of the elementary information will then be provided, along with some interesting variations you might try, and typical questions from beginners.

Second Day's Meditation Instruction

Again, the five basic steps to meditation are as follows:
1. Find a quiet place to sit where there will be few interruptions.
2. Loosen tight clothing, remove your shoes if you wish, or simply wear a comfortable robe or caftan.
3. Sit in a comfortable, relaxed position, but try not to slouch or place stress on any part of your body. Your arms should be relaxed and in your lap, on your legs, or on the arms of your chair.
4. Let your eyes close. Take two or three deep breaths and exhale slowly. Beginning with your toes, gradually relax each muscle of your body. Let your head bend gently forward, if that is comfortable. Systematically relax your toes, your feet, ankles, calves, knees, thighs, buttocks, stomach, the small of your back, your chest, your shoulders, your arms, hands, fingers, neck, facial muscles, and scalp.
5. Begin to hear your focus and let it repeat itself in your mind.

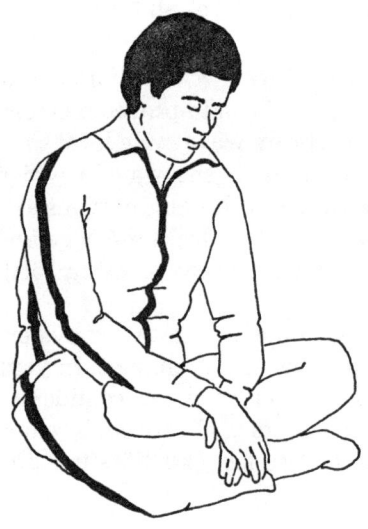

The following drawings illustrate common meditation positions which have been found to be comfortable by several meditators. I want to emphasize that a specific position is not *required* for successful meditation, but rather that these illustrations are included to aid those having difficulty. Feel free to sit or lie in any position you find comfortable and condusive to meditation.

Day 2 The Plan 47

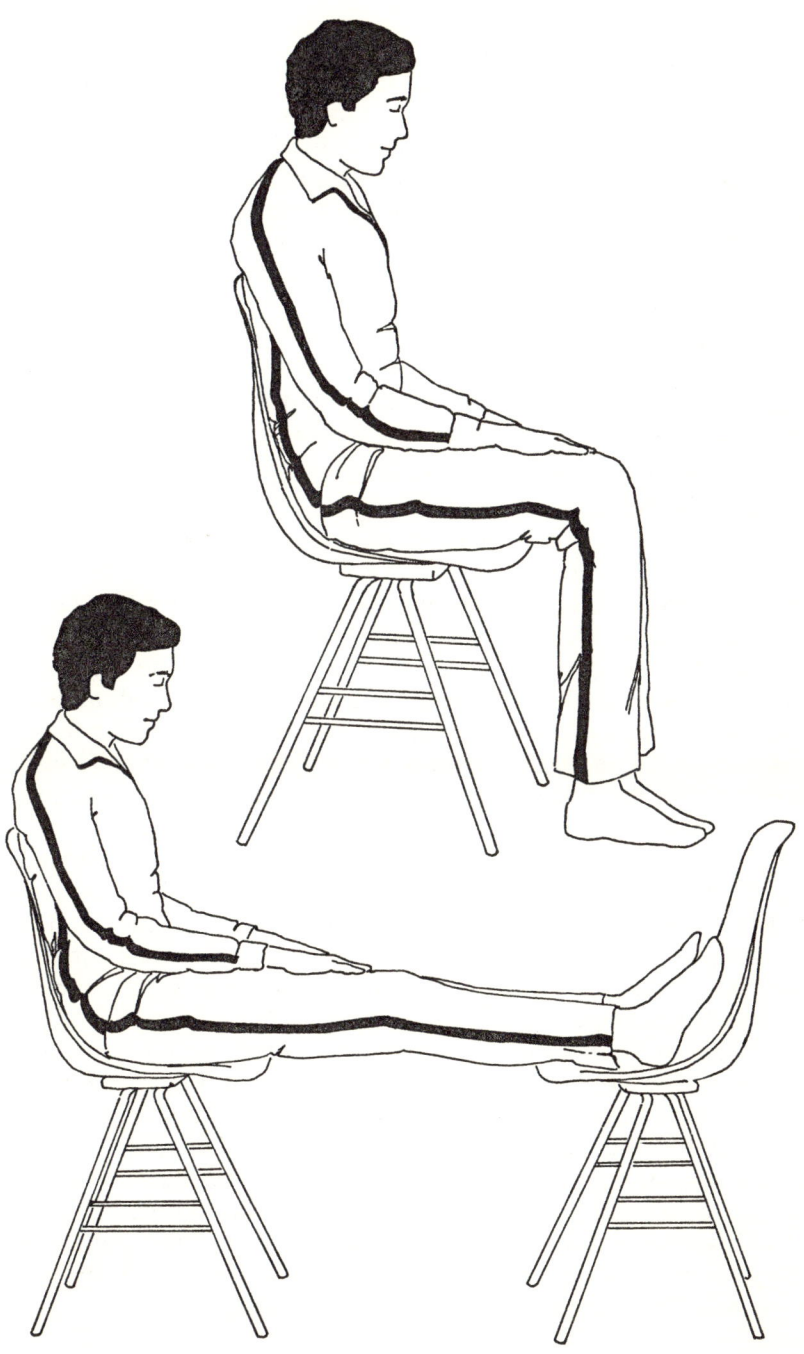

Some Interesting Variations

If you find that you are having trouble relaxing your muscles, you might try a technique that many meditators use. As you are relaxing in Step #4 (above), tighten each muscle individually as you progress, then suddenly let it go limp. It helps to think of your body as though it is getting heavier and heavier and is really putting alot of pressure on the chair underneath you. Then, as you feel completely limp, inhale and imagine that your body is lighter than air, and that you are floating right up and out of your chair.

Longfellow's words, quoted previously, ("Sit in reverie and watch the changing color of the waves that break upon the seashore of your mind") were quite illustrative of the meditation technique. His instructions can be adapted quite successfully to the process.

To use the illustrative method of meditation, follow Steps #1 through #4. Before beginning to hear your focus, draw a mental picture of yourself in a small boat in the middle of a peaceful lake. The lake gradually becomes so calm and still that there isn't even a ripple in the surface. As if by magic, you are able to slip through the bottom of the boat without harm or experiencing any discomfort. The water is very warm. Again, as if by magic, you are able to breathe under water. As you slip through the bottom of the boat, the light will diminish. As you breathe deeply, slowly let yourself sink deeper and deeper into this wonderful lake, so that the light becomes dimmer and dimmer until it is completely dark. Due to your bouyancy, you are totally weightless. Now begin to hear your focus and enter into meditation.

Another meditation enhancer is the element of controlled breathing. Many practitioners report that their rate of breathing assumes a cadence with the repetition of their focus. This is the mind and body functioning together in complete harmony. Others have noticed that their heartbeat, their breathing, and the focus are synchronous. To achieve this ideal, try the following method.

Begin by taking a deep breath and expanding your lungs laterally. Exhale just as slowly, hold for a count, then inhale. Place your hand on your wrist or throat where you can feel your pulse. Inhale to the pulse beat count of four, hold one, exhale to the count of four, hold one, then repeat. If your heartbeat is very fast, do this breathing exercise to the pulse beat of eight, holding for two beats in between breaths. Eventually, this process will be instinctual and you can do it without monitoring your pulse. Soon you will realize that your focus is in synchrony with your breathing and your heartbeat. Perfection!

Another method of enhancing the meditation experience may appeal to some. Many are enthralled with mystical pursuits and with the paranormal. They prefer to perform rites and rituals, for any number of reasons. This can be fun, if you are interested in it, and meditation can be adapted to a form of ritual as well.

Some meditators find a certain room or corner where they meditate to the exclusion of all other areas. Though this limits them in the flexibility of the technique, they like to feel as if this site has developed an aura, or special quality, and will use it only for meditation. This is fine, if that's what you're interested in.

Other people have favorite clothing or postures that facilitate their meditations. One man wraps himself in a blanket while meditating, while another woman found she had her best experiences while meditating in a warm bath. For those who are interested in the Eastern influence, you might have a "mantra" assigned to you by a T.M. teacher, and investigate the philosophical aspects associated with Eastern religions. Some people like to posture themselves in the "lotus" position common in yoga. This is beneficial since you are unable to fall or topple over while maintaining the lotus position. This is where you sit on the floor with your back straight and legs crossed. Advanced yoga students are able to place their feet on the insides of opposite thighs, near the groin area.

Any of these variations are completely all right if they appeal to you, but I must emphasize that they are not necessary to the successful practice of meditation.

Following are some typical questions and answers regarding other aspects of this program:

Questions & Answers About Meditation

QUESTION: I've heard alot about meditation, particularly Transcendental Meditation. What's so different about the meditation explained in the Total Glow program?

ANSWER: Although TM in particular has become quite popular in the United States, the form of meditation provided in this program is unique in that it uses a basic, down-to-earth approach. It does not rely on secret words or rituals, nor is supplication to a deity necessary. This method of meditation was developed from the theory that each person, regardless of lifestyle or beliefs, could realize far more of his/her own potential through exposure to the technique of meditation.

Unlike TM, this form does not require a teacher or an expensive course; you can learn all you need to know right in this book.

QUESTION: What is the major problem with those people who have trouble meditating?

ANSWER: Perhaps a major complication some people experience is that their expectations were too high in the beginning and they had disappointing results. Another aspect is that often the benefits of meditation are not immediately noticeable. It is entirely possible that you *are* benefiting, but have not yet reached the transition where it has become apparent to you. The best recommendation would be to say that each meditator should be as uncritical of progress as possible, and that they should let the benefits become known as they will.

QUESTION: Can meditation sometimes be used as a substitute for sleep?

ANSWER: No. The mental state during meditation is quite different from sleeping states. Meditation is designed to provide a feeling of restedness and refreshment which reawakens stored energy. During meditation, the mind is functioning on a more efficient level than during sleep. Also, since several hours of sleep are necessary for the restoration of energy, meditation cannot be expected to provide a substitute.

QUESTION: When is the best time to meditate?

ANSWER: There has been some debate recently regarding this question. Generally, it is best to meditate before a meal, as the body is not then involved in its digestive processes. Also, meditation is best without the complications of alcohol or drugs, which tend to be disruptive. Many people find that scheduling meditation before breakfast and before dinner acceptable. Again, you may adapt this schedule to your own needs.

QUESTION: Do I have to change my lifestyle or beliefs to practice meditation?

ANSWER: No. The method of meditating presented in this program is designed to be incorporated into anyone's schedule or lifestyle, so they need not make any changes in their normal way of thinking.

QUESTION: My work schedule is erratic. I don't want to miss any meditation sessions, but I've heard that it's best to meditate twice a day for twenty minutes each time. How can I change my meditation schedule when I need to in order to suit my working hours?

ANSWER: There aren't any rigid, inflexible rules about this method of meditation. You may meditate whenever you choose and vary the timing of each session to fit your own needs. Of course, two meditations per day of approximately twenty minutes each will provide maximum benefits for most people. But like everything else, people have differing needs. If the twice-daily meditation is impossible for you, feel free to utilize the technique in the best way you can.

QUESTION: What happens if I can't meditate for a couple of days, or just don't feel like it?

ANSWER: The important thing is to resume and continue whenever you can. Don't quit altogether because you've missed a day or two. Chances are good that you will welcome the opportunity to meditate once again.

QUESTION: I am diabetic. Is meditation safe for me and in what way can it help?

ANSWER: Meditation can help virtually everyone who is willing to try it. One of the ways in which meditation can help a diabetic is that it reduces tension and stress, which tends to stabilize the blood sugar level. This makes the control of diabetes easier.

QUESTION: Why can't I meditate more than twice a day?

ANSWER: You can, if you want to, but it has been found that twice daily is sufficient for the majority of people. Also, there is really no point in getting too much of a good thing. Like most good things, meditation can be abused by using it to escape reality, but this is certainly not recommended. It will be more beneficial to you if you think of it as the achievement of a balance between rest and action. There are certain circumstances, however, in which meditation more than twice a day can be beneficial. Pregnant women have been found to feel better by meditating more often and for longer periods of time. Also, people who are ill and confined to bed have been known to recover sooner if they meditate quite often.[2]

QUESTION: I'm seeing a psychiatrist. Will meditation interfere in any way with my psychotherapy sessions?

ANSWER: As noted earlier, many psychiatrists are recommending meditation as an adjunct to psychotherapy. There isn't any recognizable reason why meditation should interfere with your progress. See how your psychiatrist feels about it.

QUESTION: I feel that I have a dull and passive life, even though I work very hard everyday and am physically active most of the time. I want to get out of this rut, add more sparkle to my life, and feel more enthusiasm for things. What can meditation do for me?

[2]Patricia Carrington, Ph.D., *Freedom in Meditation* (New York: Anchor Press/Doubleday, 1975).

ANSWER: Although meditation isn't a quick cure-all for every problem, through deep relaxation you will gradually learn to expand your focus beyond everyday work and experiences. You will have more energy, and when you are relaxed, more of the untapped creative potential is available.

QUESTION: If a person is under sedation for an illness, is it all right to meditate?
ANSWER: It depends upon the type and strength of the medication. A particular drug may interfere with the meditative process, as will alcohol, but recent studies have shown that those hospitalized or confined to bed have meditated with very beneficial results. Check with your doctor if you have any questions, whenever you get a prescription.

QUESTION: My life is full, I'm as happy as the next person, I'm well-adjusted, and I have been very successful in my career. Do I really need to meditate?
ANSWER: Everyone can benefit from meditation; it doesn't require that a specific problem be solved, nor that a certain area needs attention. All of us have occasions of stress at some point or another, and meditation aids in dealing with it. If you meditate regularly, you will most likely notice an even greater increase in your good feelings about yourself.

QUESTION: Sometimes I have a difficult time relaxing and concentrating on my focus when I begin meditating. Thoughts keep crowding in. Why is this happening and what can I do to stop it?
ANSWER: This is normal, and there isn't any need to prevent it from happening. It simply means that your mind has been busy and that you are releasing accumulated tensions. Try not to actively concentrate on your focus; merely hear it in your mind as it comes and goes.

QUESTION: I've heard that meditation will help me become more psychic, develop ESP, telepathy, and clairvoyance. Is this true?
ANSWER: At the present time, there is no solid evidence to link the practice of meditation with psychic abilities, but studies have shown that meditation produces Alpha and Theta brain waves, wherein it is believed that most parapsychological events occur.

QUESTION: I feel like all this talk about meditation is just a passing fad. Why are so many people interested in it?

ANSWER: For several reasons. The major one is that many recognize the great need for relaxation. Another is that the mind is one of the most fascinating frontiers of research that has not yet been fully explored. What is known about the human mind is miniscule at this point, compared to the many gaps in our knowledge. People tend to be fascinated with the mind's power, whether it be recognized or not, and its untapped and undiscovered resources and abilities. Moreover, meditation deals directly with the mind's natural processes, and many researchers speculate that this trend to look inward is accelerating.

QUESTION: I have high blood pressure. My doctor tells me that I risk having a heart attack every day that I go to work. I've tried self-hypnosis, several forms of psychotherapy, and other techniques, but I still feel all wound up. Can meditation actually help lower my blood pressure?

ANSWER: Probably, if it is still in the reactive stages. High blood pressure can be caused or worsened by tension. Since you have tried these other forms of relaxation and did not experience immediate results, their benefits were probably only temporary. Some therapies are good for some people, while not-so-good for others. Meditation is a form of deep relaxation where the mind flows freely, and often it is used in conjunction with medical treatment for even more benefit. Again, check with your physician.

QUESTION: Can I do other things like housework or driving a car while meditating?

ANSWER: This is definitely not recommended. For meditation to be maximally effective, it is desirable to be in a situation where there will not be abrupt interruptions or noises. Driving *especially* requires intense concentration, and it would be best to leave meditation for another time. It *is* possible to meditate while riding in a car, however, or other form of public transportation, and many people find this an ideal time to meditate. Anything that requires even the slightest amount of attention would interfere with meditation and, conversely, trying to meditate would disrupt anything else you would be attempting.

QUESTION: After meditating, I feel as if I'm waking up from a deep sleep, but I'm not groggy. Why does this happen and is it bad?

ANSWER: It's not bad—it's good! It happens because you probably reached the Alpha brain wave level where the sense of floating can feel like sleep. Also, your muscles were as relaxed as they are when you are asleep. You are not groggy because your mind has been cleansed and is probably more alert than it has been all day.

QUESTION: When speaking about the best times for meditation, you didn't mention right before going to sleep. If meditation is so relaxing, it would seem that this would be an ideal time for it, especially for those who have trouble falling asleep. Can you explain that?

ANSWER: You're right, meditation is relaxing. But it is used to relax and calm people in preparation for other activities or situations. It isn't a good idea to meditate right before going to sleep because researchers have found that meditators who experiment with this have trouble falling alseep. One of the major effects of meditation is increased energy through relaxation. Therefore, it is usually best to use meditation early in the day and evening when you want to feel refreshed and energetic.

QUESTION: What about sex, then? Can meditating before making love improve my sex life?

ANSWER: It can. Some people who complain of a poor sex life are simply not relaxed enough to enjoy it. Meditation helps provide you with more energy and it relaxes you so that sex can be appreciated more fully. But regular practice of meditation can be more beneficial than spot meditation in this respect.

QUESTION: A friend of mine told me that I seem to be a very hostile person. What can meditation do for me?

ANSWER: Hostility often arises from fear and a confused state of mind where negative emotions have been suppressed. Meditation can help reduce the effects of this feeling. Energy can then be used in a constructive manner so that your hostility will gradually lessen. Of course, with all negative emotions, people have to allow themselves to feel them. Meditation can help you become less fearful of your emotions by allowing tension to flow out of your subconscious.

QUESTION: Why can't I say my focus out loud while meditating?

ANSWER: You can, but it takes much more effort and it is distracting. It is designed to be an inner sound, so that it can be more relaxing. It should be heard in the mind silently, rather than spoken.

QUESTION: Should I meditate before or after doing the exercises in the Total Glow program?

ANSWER: People vary in their preferences. Athletes who meditate do so before exercising because their bodies are less rigid and more limber. Try it both ways a few times so you can decide which sequence you prefer.

QUESTION: What should I do if I'm interrupted while meditating?
ANSWER: Try not to dwell too long with the interruption and simply resume where you left off. Interruptions usually don't cause any ill effects, but it's much easier when they don't occur at all. Alert your family and try to get them to understand that is is important that you are not disturbed.

QUESTION: It's in my nature to be skeptical of most things that sound out-of-the-ordinary. Are you trying to tell me that meditation is the solution to all my problems, whatever they might be?
ANSWER: No. Unfortunately, a magic solution to all problems has not yet been discovered. Meditation is simply a method that can be learned quickly, practiced easily, and it is a pleasant experience. In your particular case, meditation might serve to allow for more enjoyment of new ideas so that you can get more excitement into your life.

QUESTION: I'm really overweight, and my doctor has told me to lose weight, "or else." I've tried every diet there is, and nothing has worked to keep the weight off permanently. Can meditation help me?
ANSWER: Indeed it can, in conjunction with the nutritional aspects and exercises that make up the Total Glow program. With the exception of people who have a glandular or similar biological problem causing them to be obese, most weight problems stem from over-eating due to stress. Meditation can help you in several important ways. First, by relaxing your body and mind, you will be less anxious and will develop better self-control. Since you will be gaining an important new sense of self-esteem, it will be easier to curb your desire to over-eat. Secondly, the nutritional and exercise considerations in the Total Glow program will be of tremendous help. The recipes given are nutritious, easy, and fun to prepare, as well as being very appetizing. By replacing your current diet of fattening foods with these new dishes, your weight reduction effort will be much more pleasant. The exercises included in the program were chosen for their simplicity and body-toning qualities. In addition, you will find many suggestions for turning everyday activities into firming and toning exercises.

QUESTION: Sometimes my schedule will unexpectedly change and I don't have time to do the fifteen to twenty minutes. Can I still benefit as much from less than that?
ANSWER: Certainly. The benefits will not be as complete nor as immediate, but it will definitely be beneficial through the long-term.

The important thing is that it is best to resume full-time meditation when you can rather than stopping altogether when your schedule becomes temporarily disrupted.

QUESTION: Is spot meditation as useful as a longer one?

ANSWER: Yes, in many respects. In fact, a spot meditation session before going out for the evening can be most useful in helping you enjoy yourself. Many athletes perform spot meditation before games or matches. Also, if you have an important meeting coming up, or even a doctor's appointment, take a five-minute break beforehand and meditate. You'll find yourself much calmer and better prepared emotionally. Do continue with regular meditation sessions though, and spot meditations will be less and less necessary.

QUESTION: What are the best positions to meditate in?

ANSWER: The Total Glow form of meditation is much more flexible in this respect than other forms. You can feel completely free to sit, recline, or lie down in any position that feels most comfortable to you. I won't make suggestions because I don't want you to feel as if you "must" do it a certain way, or "must not" assume a certain position. Just try to remember that you should be as comfortable as you can be and that you need to avoid putting stress on any part of your body. In the beginning, it is probably best not to lie down, as you might have the tendency to fall asleep. Reclining chairs are favorites of many meditators, while others feel just as good lying in bed or in the bathtub.

QUESTION: I've taken an at-home course in self-hypnosis and I really like it. Will meditation interfere with this?

ANSWER: There is no reason why it should, although hypnosis and meditation are two entirely different things, with different purposes. Hypnosis is used mainly to re-condition yourself or break bad habits, although it is a form of deep relaxation. Hypnosis is also a very concentrated effort, and you are striving for specific results. Meditation, on the other hand, has no such delineated goals, and is more apt to benefit you in all respects, rather than limiting itself to one problem area. Combining the practices of self-hypnosis and meditation, however, can be very useful. When you learn to let yourself relax through meditation, it will help you accomplish successful self-hypnosis, and vice-versa. The two techniques are mutually beneficial, but I feel it is important to understand the difference.

QUESTION: I'm still not convinced that meditation is the thing for me. What else can you say to make me believe that these things will happen?

ANSWER: Try it and see for yourself! It is not my intention to try to brainwash you if you are reluctant to try meditation. If it scares you, or if you simply cannot accept it, why not do your own research and talk with some people who have tried it? Quite honestly, there is nothing about meditation that is bizarre or that can cause you any harm. Also, I obviously cannot *guarantee* that your life will change or even that you will be successful at meditating. Since all people are different, their experiences with meditation will not be identical; it will be more helpful to some than to others. I can only say that you really ought to give it a try. It is reasonably safe to say that your hesitancy due to fear about meditation will be unfounded once you've experienced the benefits.

QUESTION: Okay, I'm convinced. What do I do now?

ANSWER: Read the instructions again and try meditating. Good luck!

Exercise—It's Easier Than You Think
Why Vigorous Exercise Isn't Necessary

Exercise is something that is vitally important to every human being, and very nearly every living animal on the face of the earth. Isn't it suprising that people will give away their pets when they move to an apartment or house without a yard because, "They won't get enough exercise"? It speaks well of people's concern for the welfare of their pets, but it is amazing that they would care so much about exercise for their animals and totally neglect their own crucial need for it.

Rigorous forms of exercise, or programs that are prohibitively expensive save for the priviledged few have made people in this country shun the mere *idea* of physical activity. Those who actively pursue their own at-home, cost-free programs are few in number. If you think of it, you probably won't be able to name more than one or two acquaintances who undertake their own complete exercising routine.

A great many of us mistakenly believe that by mercilessly exercising through some sport or another on weekends, they will be physically fit. Although sports can be extremely beneficial in addition to a regular, total exercise program, this misconception couldn't be further from the truth. How many such "weekend athletes" have you seen walking around with "spare tires" and "middle-aged spread" (even if they aren't middle-aged)?

Most people have some sport or form of physical exertion they find enjoyable, whether it be golf, tennis, hiking, bowling, horseback riding, swimming, dancing, jogging, or something else. These things are fine; they're certainly better than nothing at all. But they are not enough, in and of themselves.

Dietary Habits

Any one of these activities isn't quite enough for total physical fitness. Each one is good, hard exercise (provided, of course, that you don't ride around in a golf cart while doing your nine holes), and they are of benefit to the entire body. The problem with them, however, lies in the fact that even those who participate in these activities regularly can still have major figure problems that need improvement. For example, jogging is fantastic exercise—it's good for your heart, respiratory system, legs, and will help you loose weight by burning up unused calories. But even committed joggers can still have flabby arms and pot bellies. They aren't using those muscles at all.

Another misconception that has been around for many years is the idea that dieting by itself will enable a person to lose weight and be healthy. Conversely, many believe that exercise will "make up" for over-eating. The truth remains that while both dieting and exercise will probably be good for you if you are overweight, the two must be followed in conjuction for any real progress to be made on a permanent basis. To achieve Total Glow, exercise, relaxation, and healthy eating habits must all be followed for real progress to be evidenced and maintained.

Usually, when a person goes on a crash diet (and these types of diets are not only silly, but are almost always dangerous without medical supervision), they will lose weight quite successfully at first. What most people don't realize, however, is that the weight they have lost was almost wholly comprised of water, and that the water will be right back where it came from the day the diet stops. These types of crash diets don't teach you to reform your eating habits, which is essential to weight maintenance.

Obesity and even slight heaviness is more often than not caused by water accumulation and muscles that are so out-of-shape that they cannot perform their job of supporting the body's internal organs or skeletal structure. A slouching back, not properly supported by the many muscles made specifically for this purpose, leads to an unsightly appearance. The neck droops, the rib cage sinks (giving women the appearance of sagging breasts), the stomach bulges, and the buttocks sag.

On the other hand, it is a losing battle to think that you can lose weight and inches by vigorous exercise alone, while continuing the poor habits that lead to the state in the first place. Although exercise *will* burn up calories and fat faster than simply sitting around, it is far easier to achieve your physical goals when diet and exercise are combined in a sensible program.

There are different types of exercise for different types of problems. Professional athletes (remember "Rocky"?) exercise to strengthen their muscles and build up their endurance. Ballet dancers exercise to give their bodies the flexibility and strength for demanding movements. Yoga enthusiasts exercise to unstiffen their muscles, limber their spines, and facilitate their bodily processes. All people should exercise for their own health, beauty, and well-being which leads to a better emotional outlook on life.

The human body is a remarkable mechanism and anyone who has even the slightest knowledge of the processes involved should marvel at the complexity. It is truly unfortunate that the majority of people are out-of-shape and have totally let themselves go.

Many things, especially childbirth, have been blamed for too many pot bellies. "I looked great until I had the baby," is a common excuse, but it is simply not a valid one. There are thousands of women throughout the world who have regained their youthful figures after childbirth through proper exercise. Jacqueline Onassis is a perfect example. But women aren't the only ones who need improvement in this area. By virtue of fashion, men have been hiding their weight problems under their suit coats for years, so that figure problems are not so noticeable. Through discussions with my friends and patients, however, I've learned that men really don't feel comfortable (any more than women do) about putting on weight. Sometimes they compensate for their "lost youth" through sexual conquests or by flashing money around, proving their masculinity.

What is really tragic is to see the number of teenagers who should be in perfect physical condition but are overweight and almost totally inactive. It has been theorized that a slovenly attitude is the direct result of a slovenly appearance. Activity begets activity, and when we are in good shape, we feel better and have the energy to do more things and be more involved.

The proper combination of healthful eating, relaxation, and exercise is the answer for the vast majority of adults. Unfortunately, as mentioned earlier, too many young adults fall into a neglect of their bodies just when they should be feeling most energetic and vibrant.

60   Total Glow

Through years of neglect like this, it becomes even more difficult to un-do the damage. The very least that can happen is that our appearances will suffer. The worst includes artherosclerosis, obesity, high blood pressure, and heart disease, all four of which are ultimately fatal.

How to Turn Everyday Chores Into Exercise

No matter what your age or circumstances, now is the time to begin to exercise and to start feeling better. Even the slimmest of people will benefit from exercise, due to its special ability to improve circulatory, respiratory, digestive, and mental processes.

Again, there are many ways in which to incorporate exercise into your daily routine without making your friends wonder if you are becoming "one of those health freaks." Several exercises follow which can be performed in your own home or office, and nobody will even know what you're doing.

For instance, if you are standing at a photocopier making several copies, take each one out of the tray as it is made, bend over, and place it on the floor. This bending and stretching is great for your back and thigh muscles. It will also limber you up and take out any "kinks" you might have developed from sitting for too long in one position.

The same exercise can be adapted in many ways and for several different household chores. While washing the car, try to stretch as far as possible while soaping or waxing. When you bend to re-wet the sponge or cloth, try to keep your knees straight and bend from the waist. While raking, reach out as far as possible, and pull the leaves toward you with both arms.

Vacuuming is also a great exercise, not only because it involves bending, stretching, and pulling, but because it is moderately strenous. Whenever you are standing at a counter or ironing board and must bend down for something (loading the dishwasher, for example), stand with your back straight and feet about shoulder-width apart, toes pointed out at a comfortable angle. Bend your knees and lower your body to the floor, keeping your back straight and perpendicular to the floor. Avoid the tendency to lean forward. Lower yourself slowly until you feel the need to lift your heels. Stop there and slowly raise back up. Have you ever noticed what great-looking legs ballet dancers have? This exercise is one of the reasons!

From the foregoing hints, it's easy to see how routine chores can be turned into exercises. Again, use your imagination and you're sure to come up with hundreds more.

The exercises illustrated on the following pages are to be used as a break-in to more vigorous exercises. They are very simple ones that will increase your body tone quite rapidly so that you won't have to wait long to see results. But they are not the only exercises you will need to do to achieve optimum physical fitness. Right now, stick with these exercises for a month or so, at least until you can perform them all fairly easily. Then, when you are ready to go on to more vigorous exercise, use these as a warm-up.

Both male and female models have been used to illustrate these exercises, to convey the idea that all of them can be used by either sex. Should you experience difficulty performing some of them at first, don't be discouraged. Most people find that they become quite easy after just a few days.

Remember to check with your physician before doing any exercises, especially if you have been inactive for some time.

The first group of exercises are to help limber, tone, and strengthen your back muscles. Your back gets alot of abuse through the years, and is a prime target for fatigue, ache, and other problems.

Exercises to Help Your Back

The Cobra

This exercise will strengthen your back muscles, and help maintain flexibility in your neck and upper back.

Lie face down on the floor with your hands palms downward at shoulder level, fingers pointing toward those of your other hand.

As you inhale, slowly raise your upper body, as if you are inching up one vertebra at a time. Try not to push with your arms until you have raised up with your back as far as possible. Then push gently with your arms to bend back as far as possible. Arch your neck and look toward the ceiling.

As you exhale, slowly lower your body again using your back and not your arms.

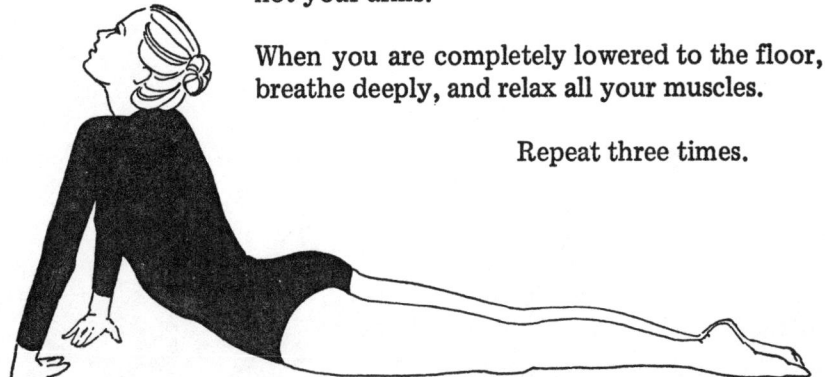

When you are completely lowered to the floor, breathe deeply, and relax all your muscles.

Repeat three times.

The Elephant Walk

If you frequently have discomfort or pain in your lower back, this exercise will help alleviate it by stretching the muscles involved. It is also great for firming and toning the muscles in the back of your thighs.

Stand with your feet about a foot apart, bend from the waist and, with knees bent as much as necessary, touch your fingers to your toes. Inhale and straighten your right leg, then exhale and relax. Inhale and straighten your left leg, then exhale and relax. Perform this exercise five times for each leg.

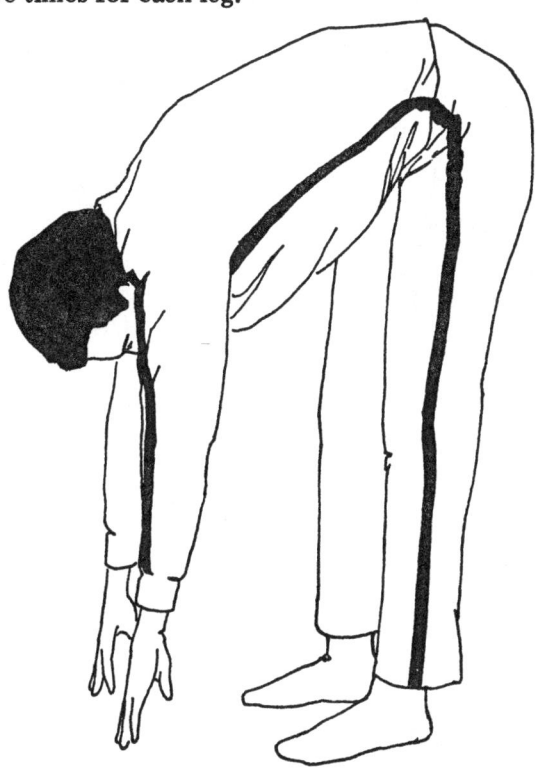

Shoulder Tension Reliever

If you have been sitting hunched over for too long, or if your back is suddenly uncomfortable, this exercise is bound to provide relief. Over the long term, it will also help correct round shoulders, and improve flexibility.

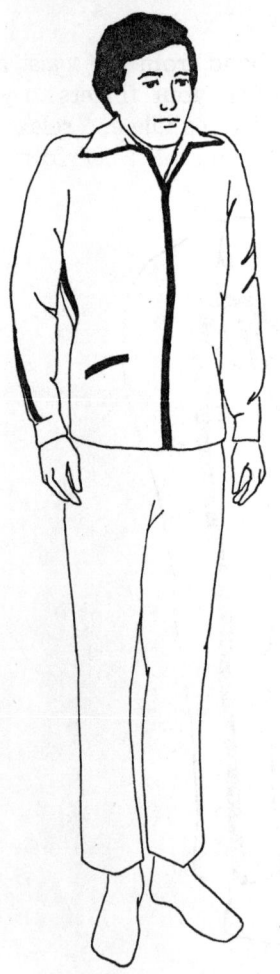

Stand or sit upright with shoulders back, down, and relaxed. Slowly, and in one continuous motion, swing your shoulders back, down, front and up. Continue to do this exercise until you feel the easing of tension in your shoulder blade area.

Arm Swings

This exercise is great for getting the circulation going in your arms and relieving "writer's" or "accountant's" cramp. It's also a good "wake up" exercise when you are feeling tired or need to clear your mind.

Stand upright with your feet about a foot or two apart, with your arms crossed in front of your chest. As you inhale deeply, swing your arms out and back as far as you can. Exhale, and swing them to the front. Continue doing this exercise four or five times whenever you feel the need, and try to make it one, fluid movement.

Exercises for Your Stomach, Waist, and Abdomen

Next comes a group of exercises that also benefit the back, but will effectively tone and trim the stomach, waistline, and abdomen.

Inverted Bend

Not only does this exercise strengthen your back, it is great for buttocks and stomach muscles. Take it slowly the first few times.

Lie on your back, knees bent and feet about a foot apart, flat on the floor. Your arms should be straight and at your sides. Slowly tighten your buttocks and lift your hips off the floor. Try to raise as high as you can, then hold for a count of five. Release and lower your hips to the floor slowly. Repeat five times.

Day 2 The Plan 67

Sledge Hammer

While performing this exercise, try to make your movements as continuous and fluid as possible. The benefits include adding flexibility to your spine, slimming the waistline, toning and firming the back thigh muscles.

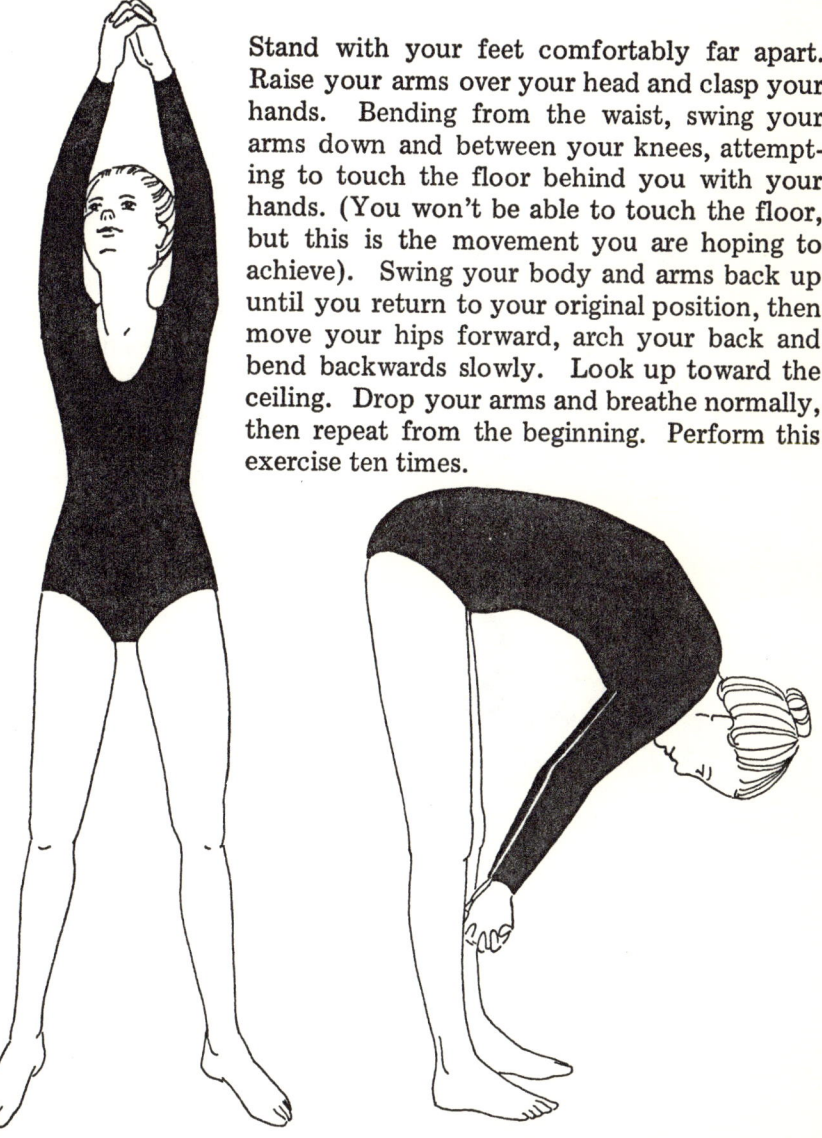

Stand with your feet comfortably far apart. Raise your arms over your head and clasp your hands. Bending from the waist, swing your arms down and between your knees, attempting to touch the floor behind you with your hands. (You won't be able to touch the floor, but this is the movement you are hoping to achieve). Swing your body and arms back up until you return to your original position, then move your hips forward, arch your back and bend backwards slowly. Look up toward the ceiling. Drop your arms and breathe normally, then repeat from the beginning. Perform this exercise ten times.

The Half-Locust

This exercise will strengthen your back, arm, and leg muscles while stretching the hamstrings.

Lie face down with your hands in fists by your sides, backs of hands on the floor. Place your chin forward on the floor. Your legs should be straight with your feet together and toes pointed.

As you inhale, raise your right leg as high as you can without rolling over to the left or bending your knee. Hold your right leg up in this position for a count of five, then exhale as you lower it back to the floor. Take a few deep breaths, then repeat with your left leg. Do each leg three times.

(After a while, you might be inclined to try FULL LOCUST, where you raise *both* legs simultaneously. This however, is not an exercise for beginners.

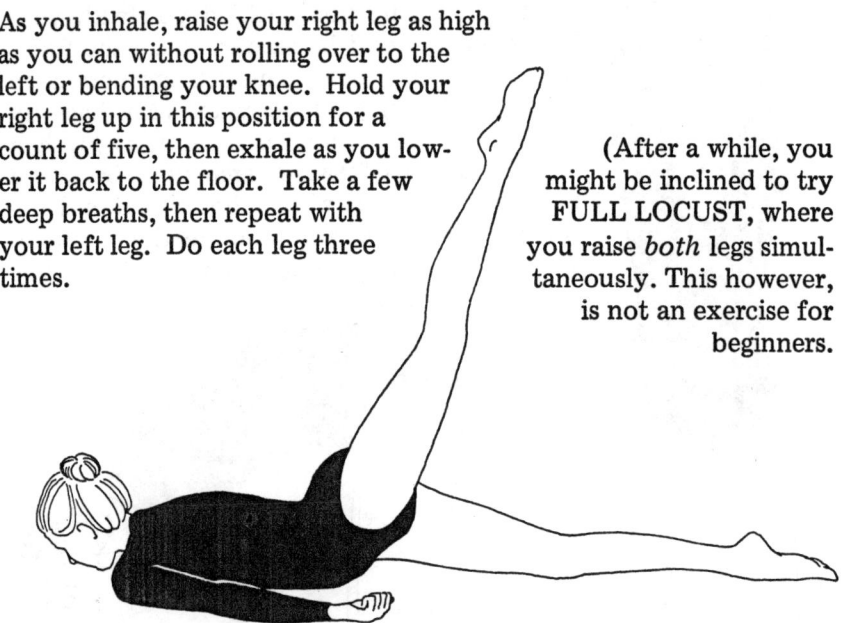

The Bow

This exercise is good for almost every part of your body. It will firm your abdomen, strengthen your back, tone your arms and legs. It's not as easy as it looks, but very beneficial, once you get the hang of it.

Lie face down with knees bent and legs raised. Reach back with your arms and grasp your ankles. As you inhale, raise your knees and head simultaneously. Push your feet firmly against your hands to lift your knees and head as high as you can. Hold for a count of five. Exhale while slowly lowering your head and knees to the floor. Repeat three times.

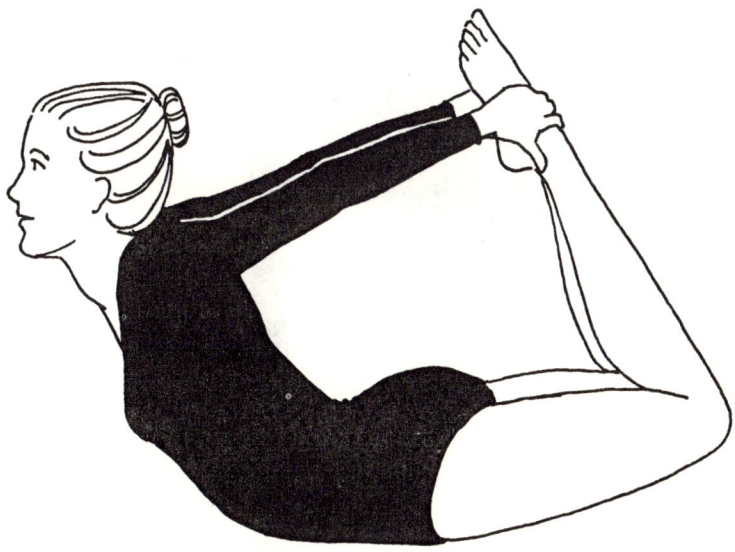

The Triangle

At first, this might look like an exercise left over from high school gym class. It is similar, but it is performed very slowly, rather then in a swift, bouncing motion. It is a great exercise for firming the waist and stomach, stretching the muscles in the legs, and toning the muscles in your upper arms.

Stand with your feet as far apart as they will go. Slowly raise your arms straight out at your sides until they are shoulder level. Inhale as you *slowly* bend to the left until your left hand grasps your left ankle. Bend directly to the side, not the front. Your right arm should swing over your head in a wide area until the inside of your elbow is touching your ear. Hold for a count of ten. Exhale while returning to original position, and repeat on the other side.

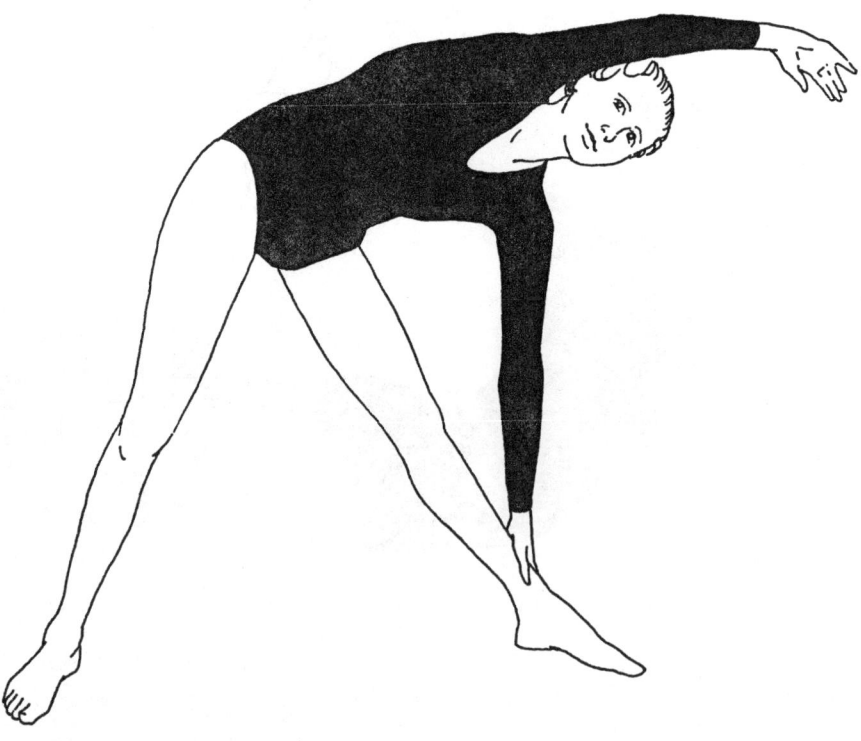

The Plough

This is one of the best exercise for overall conditioning. It firms the stomach and strengthens the back, while stretching and toning arms and legs.

Lie on your back with your arms at your sides and your legs straight together. Slowly raise both legs off the floor and swing them back over your head.

Lower your legs so that your toes touch the floor, and point them toward your head as much as possible. Keep your knees straight. Hold for twenty seconds, then slowly raise your legs up, lower them, and return to your original position.

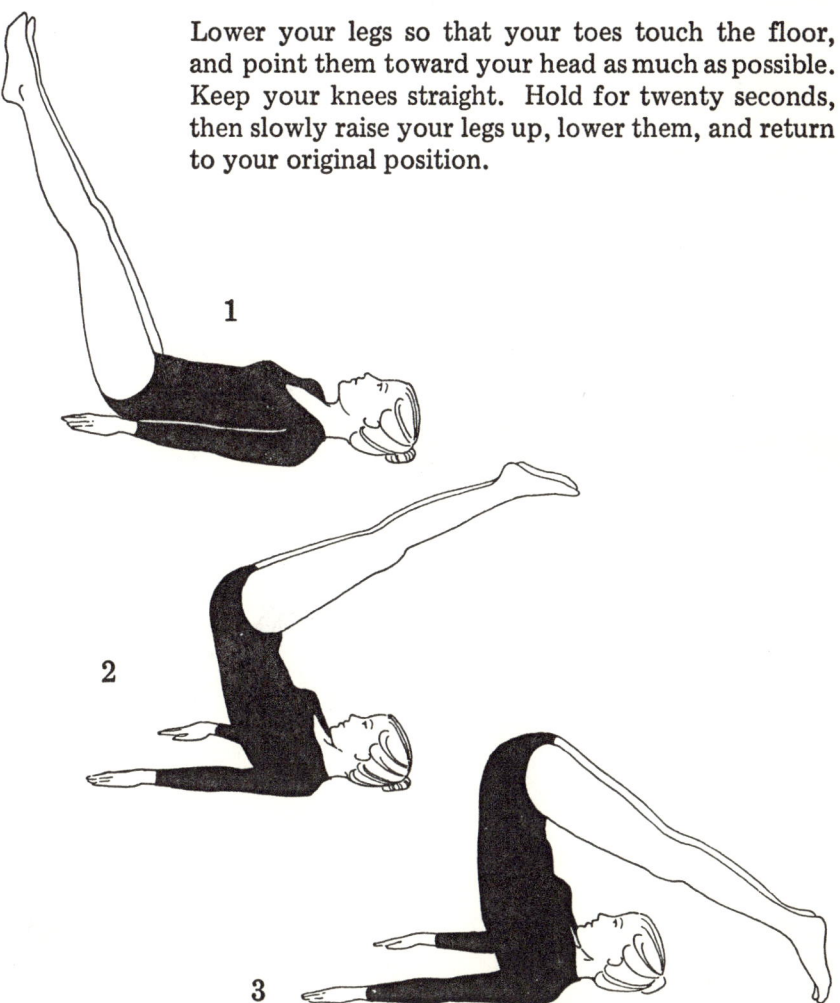

Sit Ups With A Chair

This may look like it's more difficult than standard sit-ups, but actually it's not. It's easy, and once you have mastered this, you can start with regular, flat-on-your-back sit ups.

Place your heels on a chair seat, couch, or side of your bed. Inhale and raise up rolling each vertebra off the floor one by one. Touch your toes and start back down. On the way back, lower yourself as slowly as possible, keeping your arms outstretched in front of you and your chin down. The more often you do this exercise, the better at it you will become. There's no better exercise for firming the stomach and abdomen.

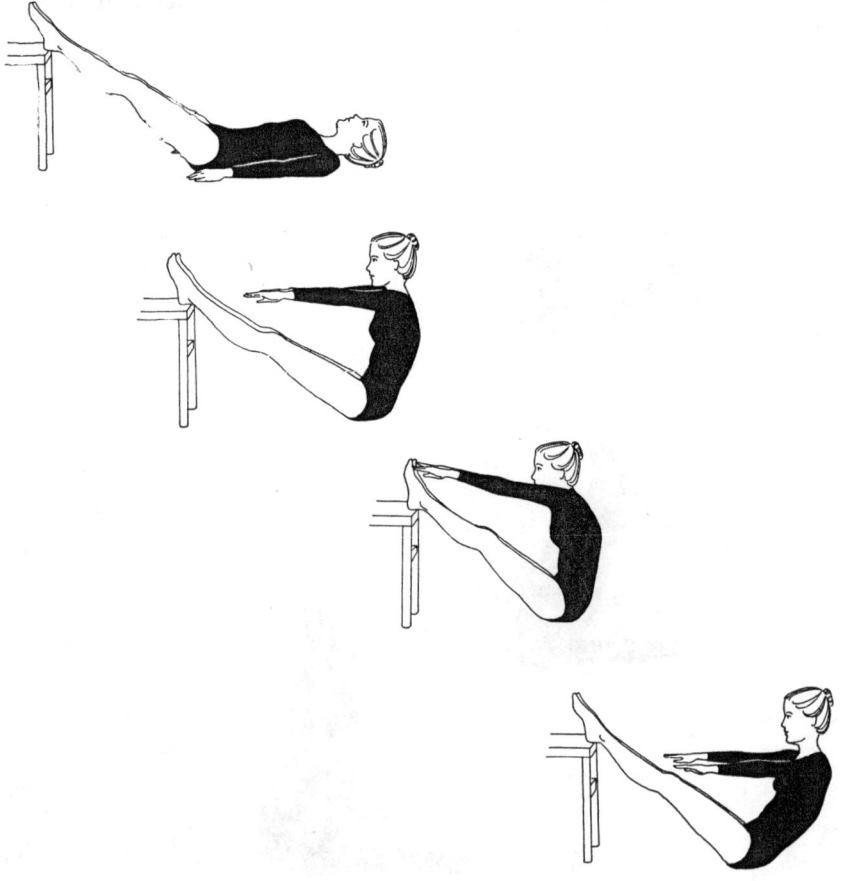

Semi Sit Ups

This exercise has a double benefit. Not only does it tend to tone the muscles in the neck and throat (where double chins develop), but it also firms the abdomen.

Lie on your back with your hands at your sides. Inhale, and tighten the stomach muscles while at the same time lifting your head and shoulders off the floor. Hold this position for the count of five, then release. When your abdomen gets a little stronger, you might want to try lifting your feet off the floor while raising your head and shoulders.

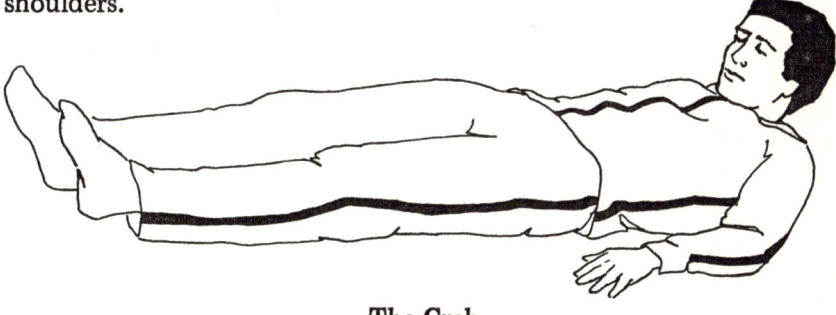

The Crab

Miraculous results can be obtained through the application of this exercise. It will effectively pare inches from your waistline and greatly strengthen your stomach muscles.

Lie on your back with your knees bent to a comfortable angle. With hands behind your head and fingers entwined, inhale and tighten your abdominal muscles. Lift your head and shoulders from the floor, then increase the abdominal pull and lift both feet off the floor. Count to five, then release.

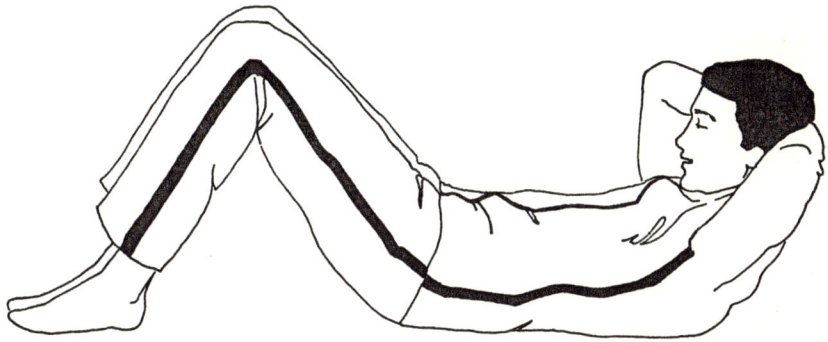

Scissor Kicks

This exercise will appear difficult at first, especially if your abdominal muscles are untoned. Keep trying, though, and soon you will develop a beautifully firmed stomach. This exercise also adds flexibility and tone to the inner and outer thighs.

Lie on your back with your arms at your sides, about a foot from your body. Lift your legs together to a position that is approximately a 45 degree angle from the floor. Spread your legs out as wide as you can, then bring back together, crossing them in scissor fashion. Spread again, and cross again with the opposite leg going under the other one. Perform this exercise five times.

Rib Cage Lifts

This exercise's waist-whittling qualities will make this one a favorite!

Sit cross-legged on the floor, arms relaxed on knees. One at a time, lift each arm overhead and reach as high as you can, as if you are lifting your rib cage right off your waist. Tilt you head back and look up to the ceiling each time. Lower your arm and repeat with other arm. Perform five times each side.

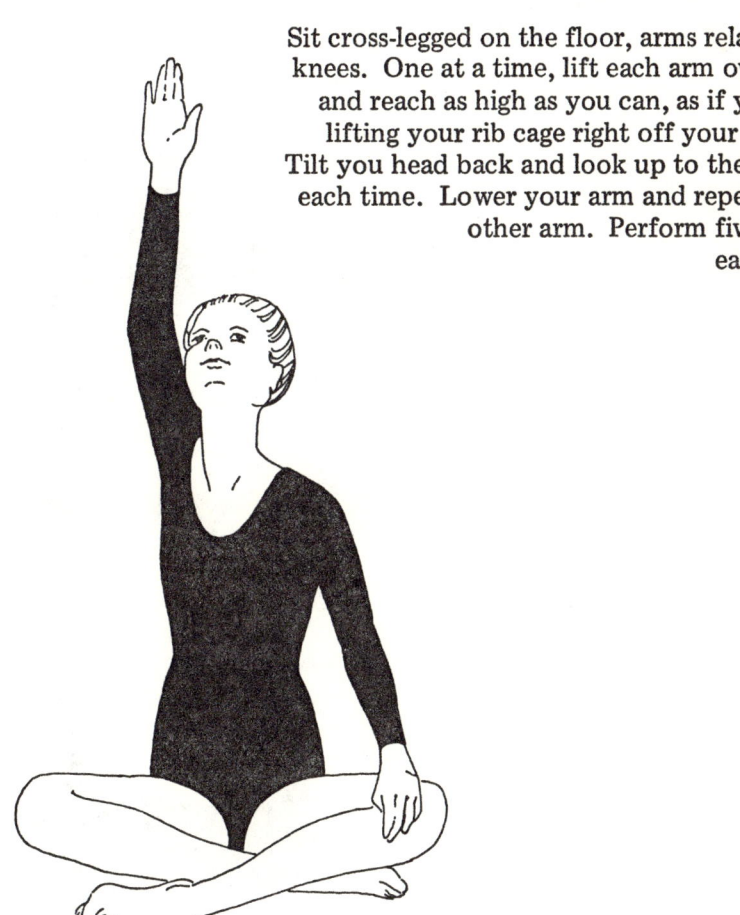

Exercises for Your Legs

The next exercises are primarily for the legs, where most of us begin to develop fat deposits early in life.

Arc Angels

This a common exercise for a very good reason. It firms the buttocks and hips, thighs, and flexes the spine.

Kneel on all fours, knees about a foot apart. Slowly raise your right knee and drop your head so that your knee and chin almost touch. Swinging your legs back and out, straighten and raise as high as you can, while tilting your head back and arching your back. Repeat three times for each leg.

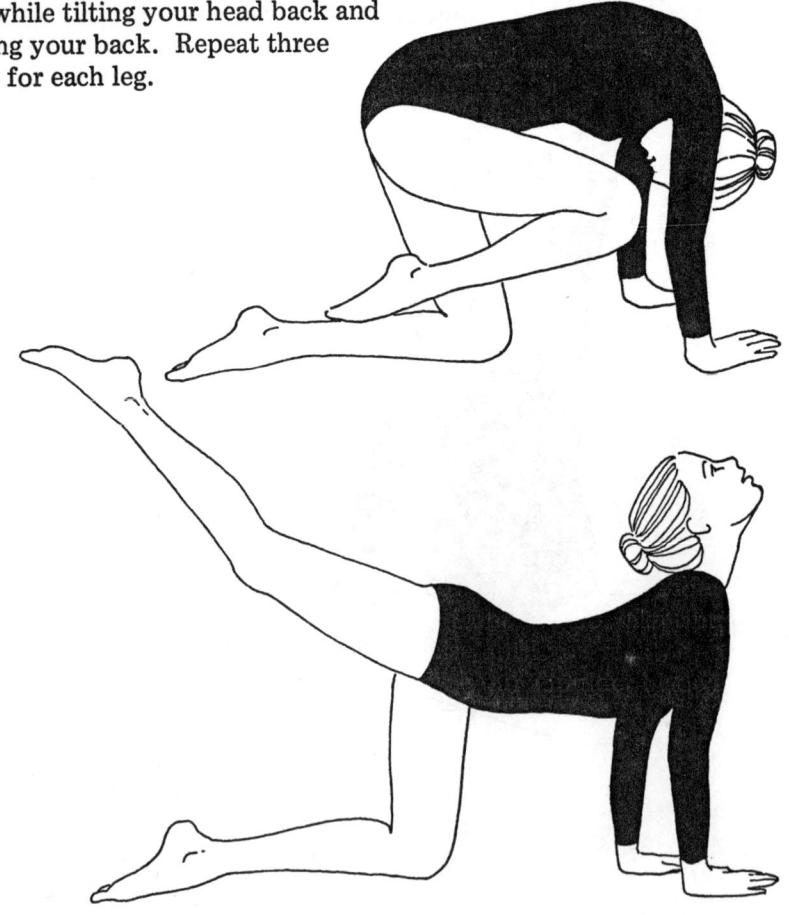

Day 2 The Plan 77

The Hamstring Stretch

This exercise is especially good for toning and firming the inner thigh region.

Sit on the floor, with your knee bent and curled underneath so that your foot rests beneath your left thigh. Support yourself by placing your right arm on the floor behind you. Bend and raise your left leg and grasp your left foot with your left hand in the instep area. Gently try to straighten your left leg and hold it for a count of ten. If your leg will stretch out straight, don't lock your knee, but gradually flex your leg out straight. If your knee has a tendency to lift off the floor, concentrate on pressing the knee into the floor.

Repeat on right side, flexing your leg bent and straight until eventually you can hold your leg out straight.

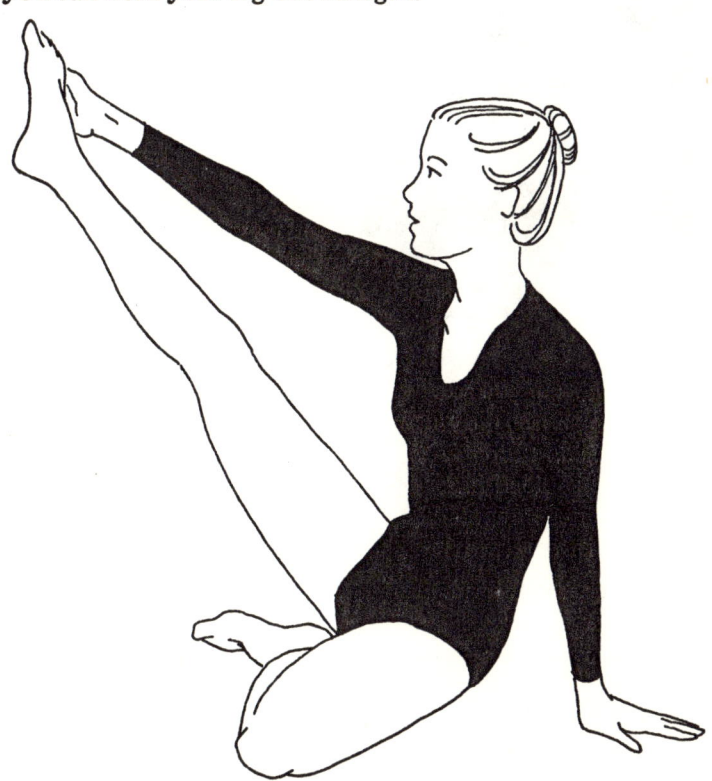

The Swashbuckler

This exercise is performed in a gentle, swinging motion from side to side. Not only is it fantastic for the inner thighs and calves, but will help develop poise and coordination.

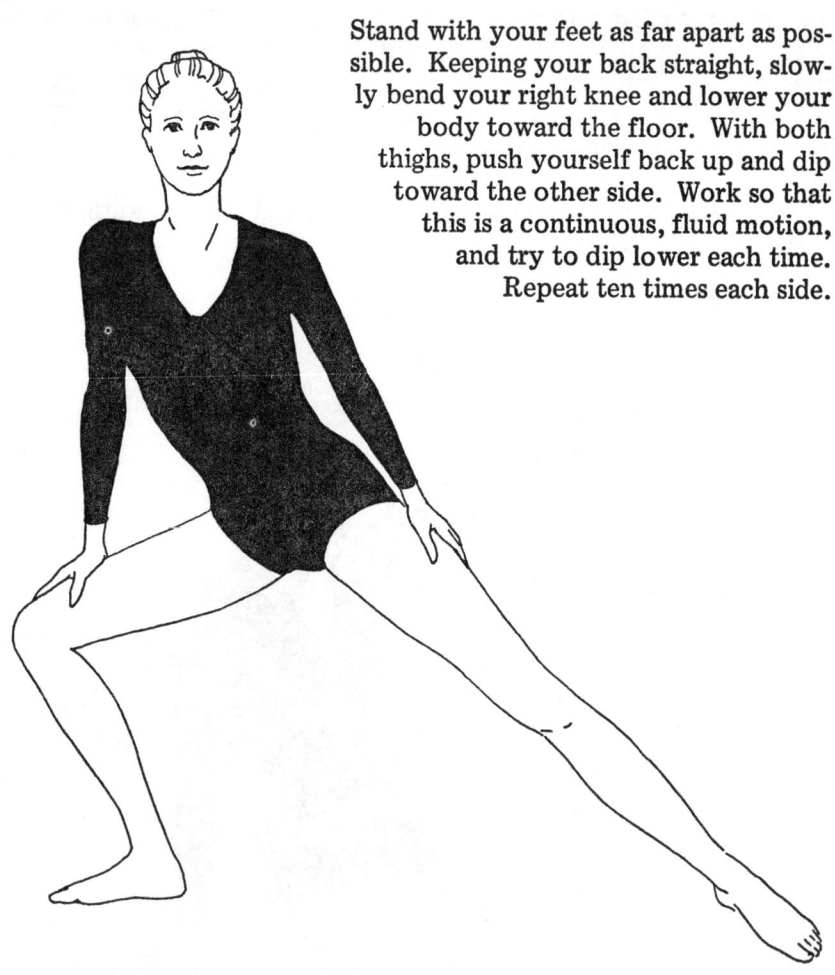

Stand with your feet as far apart as possible. Keeping your back straight, slowly bend your right knee and lower your body toward the floor. With both thighs, push yourself back up and dip toward the other side. Work so that this is a continuous, fluid motion, and try to dip lower each time. Repeat ten times each side.

Bottom Lifts

This exercise is not as easy as it looks, so be careful to do it properly for full benefit. It will strengthen thigh muscles, and firm the buttocks.

Place yourself in a position where you are sitting on your heels, your back is perfectly straight, and your hands are resting on the small of your back. Keeping your back straight, head back, and buttocks tucked in, slowly raise your body to a kneeling position, then inch-by-inch return to sitting.

Do about five times, then stretch your legs out straight and relax.

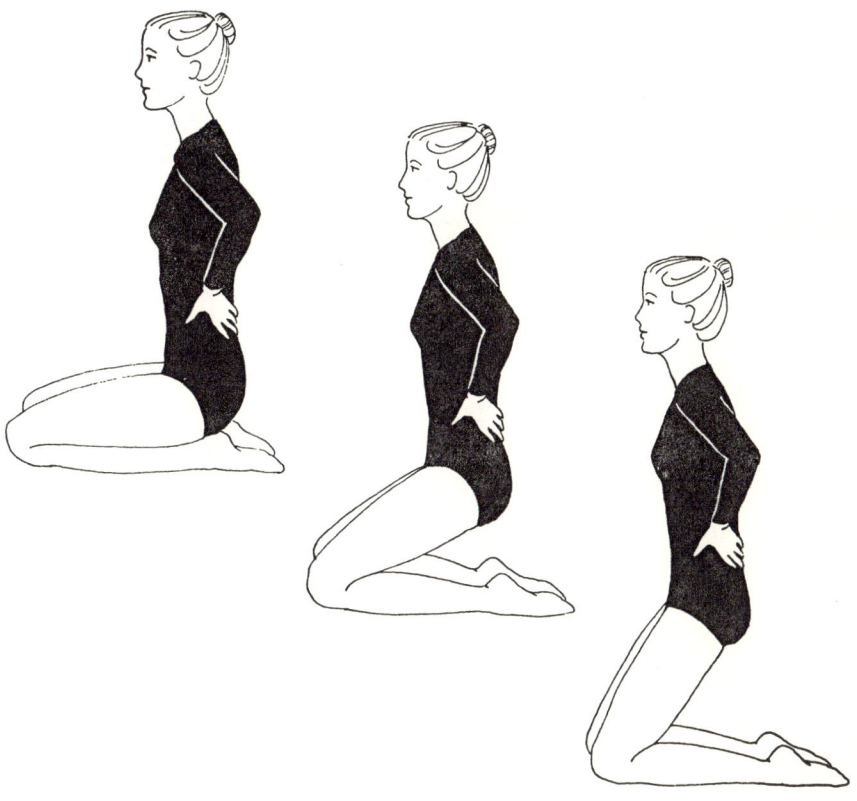

Rockettes Kicks

Due to inactivity and sitting for long periods of time, the legs tend to get stiff and circulation slows down. This exercise not only "wakes up" your legs by getting the circulation moving again, but also serves to stretch important muscles and add flexibility.

Stand by the side of a chair or desk, with your right hand on the back of the chair for support. Inhale and swing your left leg forward and up, kicking as high as you can. At first, you may bend your right knee a little, but later work toward keeping it straight. As you exhale, swing your leg back and up. Continue this movement several times, then turn around and repeat for the other leg.

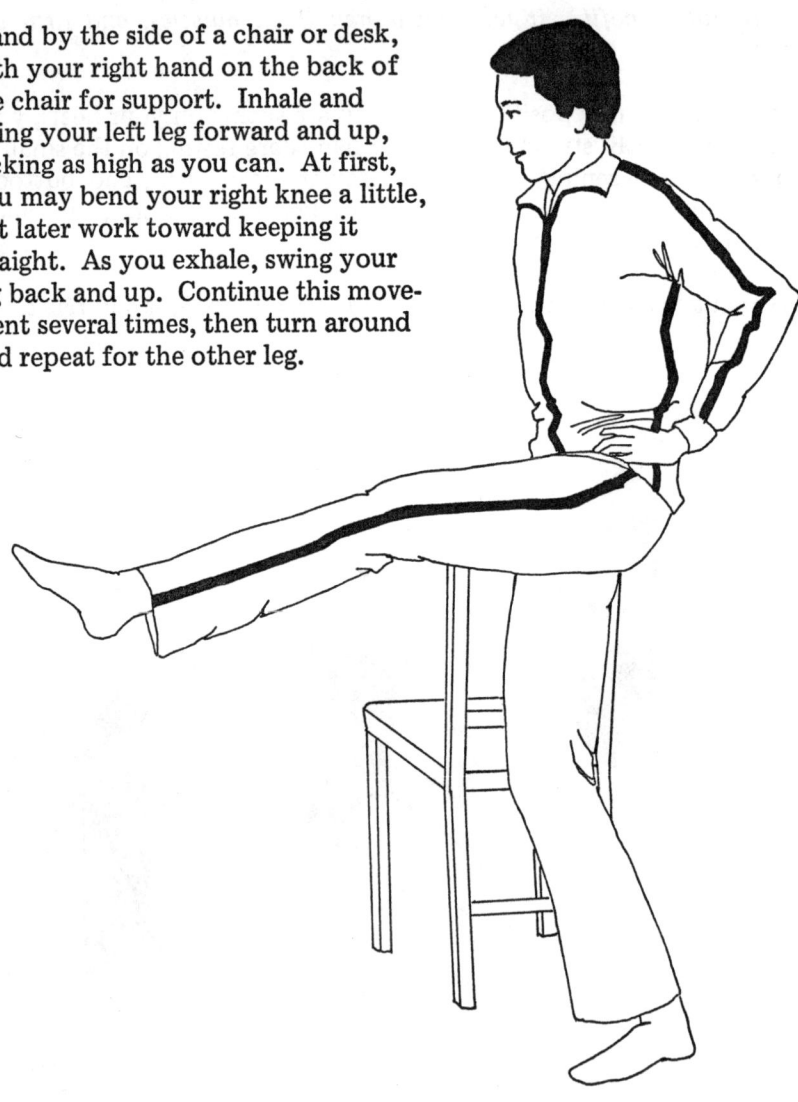

Toe Raises

While appearing quite simple at first glance, this exercise is marvelous for your calves, ankles, and thighs. You will feel this immediately, and it will tone and firm very quickly. Always perform this exercise before jogging.

Stand erect with your feet about four inches apart, toes resting on a rather thick book, heels on the floor. Rapidly, raise up on your toes, then lower. On the way down, do not let your heels touch the floor.

Perform this exercise ten times in rapid succession. Then rest and shake your legs.

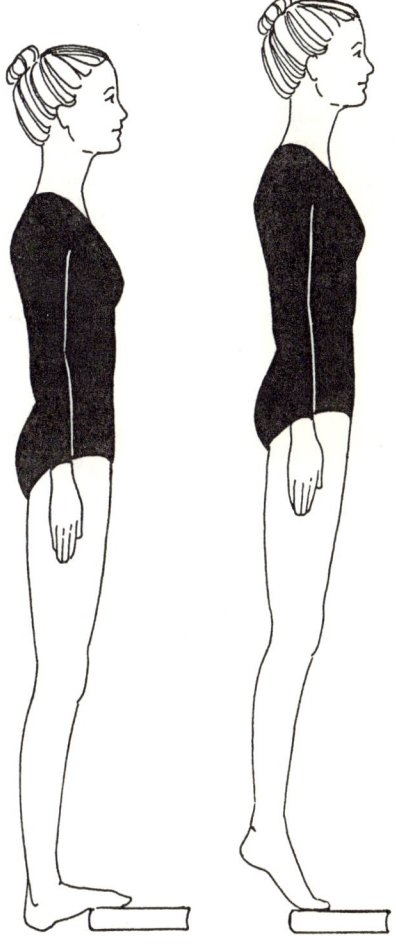

Exercises for Specific Areas

The following set of exercises deals more with specific figure and body-area problems.

Double Chin Chasers

A double chin is unfortunately, one of the first signs of age. The body has been fighting the pull of gravity for many, many years, and most often, the soft tissue under the chin is the first to succumb to the force. Luckily, there is a very simple exercise to combat this event, or to prevent it's ever taking place.

Sit at your desk (or table) with your elbows on the desk. Make a fist with your left hand, and cup the fingers of your right hand over it. Rest your chin on your hands and try to open your mouth, while resisting with your hands. Hold for the count of ten.

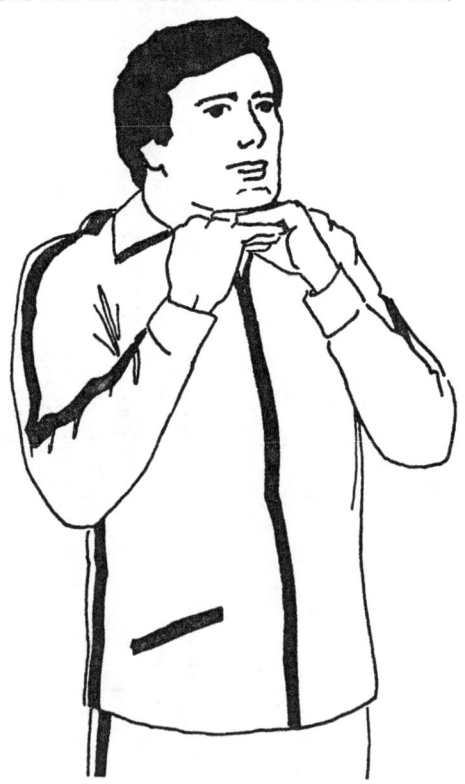

Swing Strengtheners

For this exercise, you will need a broom, rake, mop, or some other object of similar dimensions and weight. Doing this exercise once a day will greatly improve the strength in your arms, and will therefore improve your tennis stroke or golf swing.

Stand with your feet about shoulder-width apart. Grasp the broom handle in your left hand and slowly raise the broom up to shoulder level. Repeat with the other arm. Make sure to keep your arm straight!

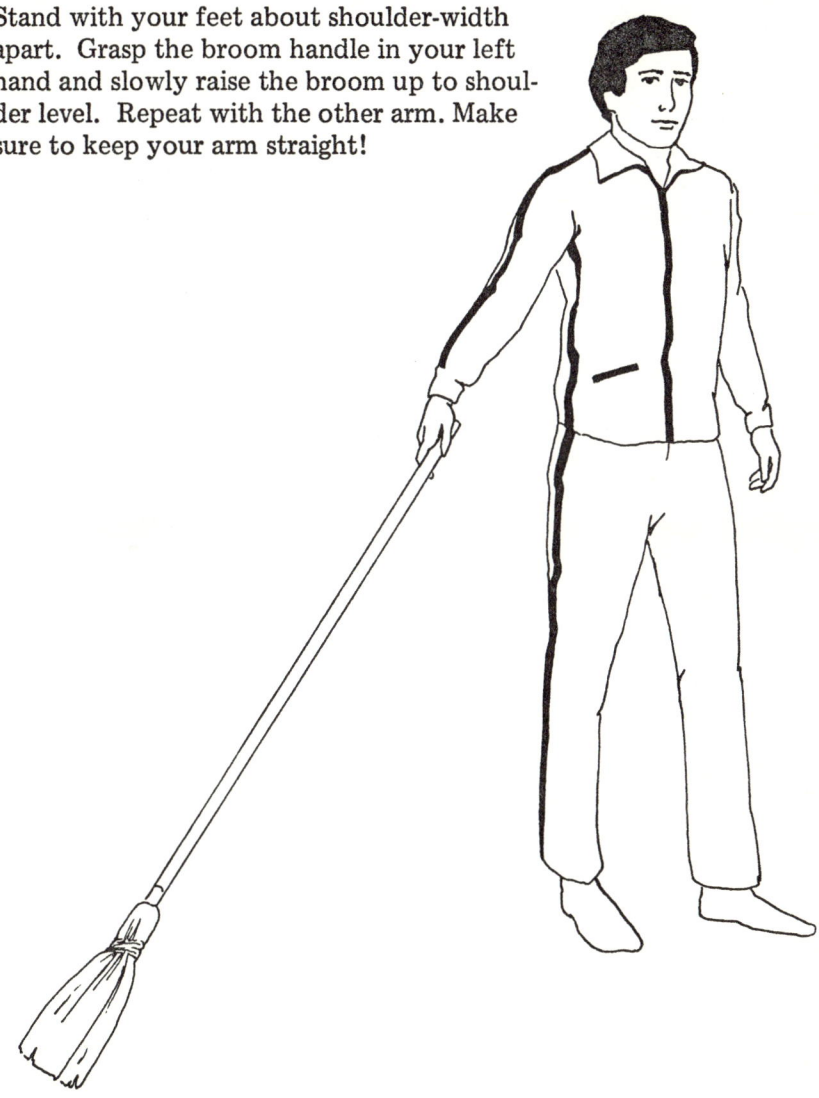

Pre-Jogging Stretch

This exercise is essential in preparation for jogging or walking. It is also good as a morning stretch, to get the circulation going in your legs, or to ease tired feet and ankles.

Stand facing a wall at arms's length, feet slightly apart, toes pointing toward wall. Place both hands flat on wall surface at shoulder height and slowly lean in toward the wall, bending elbows. Lean in until you can feel the pull in calves and tendons in the backs of your ankles, then push back with arms. Repeat ten times before jogging.

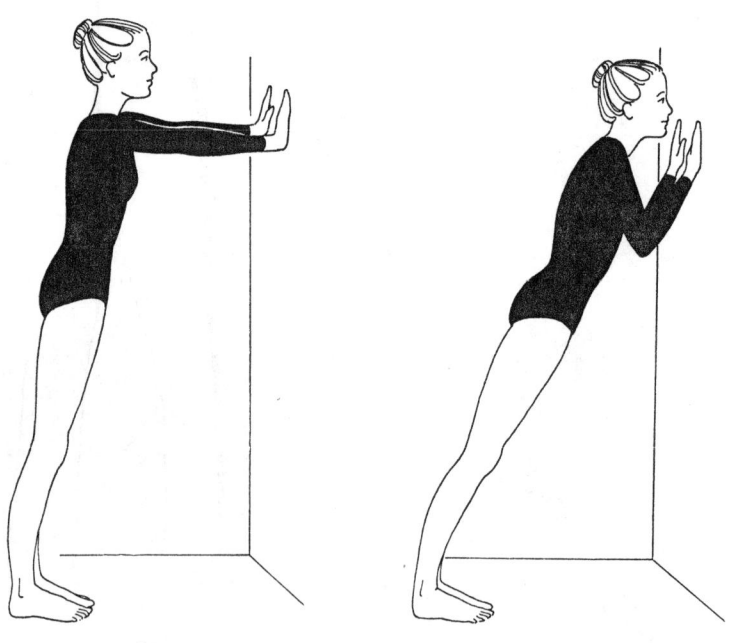

Thigh Trimmers

People who work in offices where they are sitting all day find this exercise especially beneficial. It strengthens muscles in inner and outer thighs, flexes the spine, and firms leg muscles in general.

Lie on your back, arms spread out straight at shoulders, feet together and legs straight. Swing your right leg up and over your body, attempting to touch your left hand with your foot. Try to keep hips on the floor. Slowly swing leg back, up, and down to original position. Repeat with other leg. Perform five times on each side.

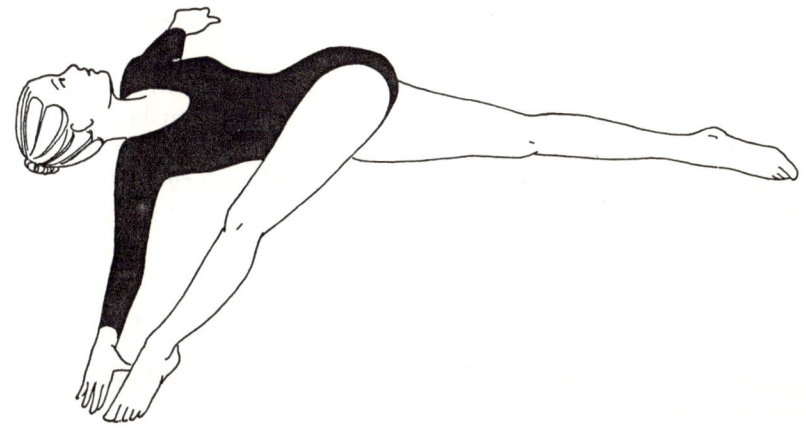

Knee Pull Ups

This is a good exercise for firming thighs and easing lower back pain.

Lie on your back, legs straight and feet together. Slowly bend right leg, bringing knee up to your chest. Wrap arms around your leg, gently pulling your knee toward your chest. For extra benefit to stomach and back muscles, bring your head up and touch forehead to knee while pressing leg to chest. Repeat for other leg. Perform this exercise five times on each leg.

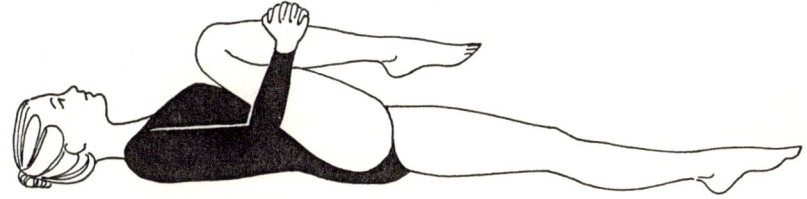

Aerobics

The approach thus far has been planned to help get you started with exercise. Many of these have been designed to help tone the skeletal muscles. As mentioned, so many people try more strenuous physical activities only to become discouraged because of the difficulty of following through, or because they developed painfully sore muscles.

Some of the more vigorous "aerobic" exercises, however, can be beneficial if you approach them correctly and your physical condition permits. It is vitally important to get your doctor's okay. Your cardiovascular system is made up of vital organs that are crucially important to your health. By gradually introducing and increasing the pace and time spent in aerobic activity, you strengthen your cardiovascular system.

Our bodies are designed to be more like marathon runners than the relatively sedentary people most of us are. My husband has lowered his heart rate from seventy to fifty-two beats per minute in a two-year period. This has been accomplished to a large extent by jogging three miles three times a week and by playing tennis the other three or four days.

I suggest, however, that you wait at least six months after being on the Total Glow plan before beginning an aerobic exercise program. It is important to let the many positive benefits of both muscle tone and nutrition be in effect. If you don't wait before attempting more strenuous exercises, you may add an unhealthy level of stress to your body. The reason for this extra word of caution is that, unfortunately, most of us are in a far worse condition than we realize.

The toxicity of our environment (including our food and water), and the pace and stress of modern living have combined to take a severe toll on our overall health. Therefore, even if you feel up to it, it's wise to get yourself into better shape before you try any form of strenuous exercises.

The best, most convenient, and most efficient forms of aerobic exercises are: jogging, cycling, swimming, and walking. Other sports, especially ones like tennis, handball, racquetball, and paddle tennis can also be quite helpful. However, they are not as efficient and are far more difficult to measure in terms of their effectiveness. Each person is at a different level of ability, causing great variations in the amount of exercise each one receives. If you enjoy these sports, by all means participate in them, but I cannot break them down into their worth or benefit, so my discussion will center around the first ones I mentioned.

The factor common to all aerobic exercise, when performed correctly, is the continuous, gentle pressure on the heart and lungs. You can engage in any one of them at any age, providing, of course, that your condition and general level of health permits doing so.

Here are some tips in getting started with aerobic exercises:

1. Jogging—Invest in a good pair of jogging shoes. This will help prevent foot, leg, or back aches, shin splints, and other problems. Wear heavy wool or cotton socks and comfortable clothes. Even after you get your doctor's okay, take it very easy in the beginning. Jog/walk no more than 12 minutes a day for the first week. As you jog, be sure you don't let yourself get out of breath enough so that you are unable to speak in a normal conversational voice without gasping for breath. If you get pains in your side, stomach, or chest, stop jogging and walk quietly for a quarter mile or so. Don't stop suddenly or sit down. You must keep your body moving since you will then have less of a chance of heart attack, muscle cramps, or other problems. Your body needs to gradually "wind down" much the same way that a race horse does after a race.

In a week or two (or possibly a month or two, depending on your condition), you can increase your jogging time to fifteen minutes. There's no rush to get to this point, so listen to your body and let it tell you when you are ready to go on to more time. By gradually increasing your time by three minutes each week, you will soon be able to jog for twenty to thirty minutes at least four times a week. I feel that it's more important to measure results in time rather than in distance, but if you want to measure your distance, drive over a course with your car and use the speedometer to measure it.

You will be able to jog comfortably in all types of weather, except when the temperature drops below 10° F. or goes beyond 90° F. If you live in extremely hot or cold climates, you may be able to locate a gym or indoor track. You can also jog in place, but for many people this can become boring. Try it and see if you like it before discounting it altogether, though.

When it's cold, you'll be surprised how comfortable you feel when you wear appropriate clothing. At the minimum, you'll need a hat that covers your ears, gloves, and a warm jogging suit. Add a sweater, your jogging shoes, and warm socks.

In warm temperatures, wear light clothing—shorts (light cotton is best, since it "breathes"), a tee shirt or tank top, and shoes and socks. Running in a gentle rain or light snow can be lots of fun. I never would have believed it until I tried it the first time. In a thunder storm, however, it is wise to get indoors as soon as possible.

Usually, it's a good idea to carry enough money in coin to make a phone call in case you get stuck away from home and need someone to come pick you up. Some joggers carry small plastic water bottles with them to quench their thirst on distance runs.

The type of running surface and location chosen will make a big difference. In the beginning, if you have a cinder quarter-mile track available or a grass covered field, it would be wise to jog there. These surfaces will be easier on your feet, legs, and back because they are softer than running on sidewalks or macadam.

After a period of time, when your physical condition improves, try running on sidewalks or alongside the road. If you are running beside the road surface, always jog facing traffic. I like to change the location of my jogs just for variety, although some of my friends have enjoyed running on the same track for years. Find out which method you prefer.

Some long-time joggers report a form of self-hypnosis that can occur while running around a track, while others get bored. To me, the greatest place to jog is through a beautiful country setting. A city jog can also be fun as you learn the streets, houses, and office buildings better. Look for trees along the way and try to become familiar with them, identifying them for added interest. For me, running around a track gets monotonous after awhile, but you are better able to gauge your progress and distance this way.

The time of day to jog varies with each individual as to his or her schedule, lifestyle, and whether or not they are "morning" or "night" people. You may want to vary your jogging times as I do. Anytime is all right, as long as you wait for about two hours after a big meal. If you jog at night, be sure to wear light-colored clothing and a reflective vest so that you will be easily seen by drivers. Sporting goods stores sell the vests, and reflective stripes that you can stick onto your back, chest, and shoes.

When you get into more frequent and regular jogging on hard surfaces, your shoes will wear out fairly quickly. A marathon runner can wear shoes down badly in just one race. I've found that using a product called "Shoe Goo" on the spots which wear the most can greatly prolong the life span of the heels and add stability to the shoes. "Shoe Goo" is available in most sporting goods stores.

Jogging is the most efficient aerobic exercise in the sense that it takes less time than any other exercise. A person of any age can engage in it, if they are physically able. It involves less equipment and facilities—all you need is a pair of running shoes. Some individuals, however, do not enjoy it, nor do they gain a sense of well-being and pleasure after jogging. If you are this type of individual, don't put yourself down as a failure, and try not to be discouraged.

Some people simply dislike the whole idea of jogging and do not respond well to it. They look upon it as a sense of drudgery. If you feel this way, after making an attempt to appreciate it, try not to be too disappointed. If you don't develop a sense of enjoyment and accomplishment with jogging, it's probably best to forget it and try some other form of aerobic exercise. The other alternatives may be more to your liking, and the effects are approximately as favorable.

2. Cycling—Even if you haven't been on a bicycle since childhood, you can have lots of fun and achieve better health through renewing your interest. A bicycle is ideal for people with many different back conditions which do not allow them to jog. A good 10-speed bike is a good investment in your future health, and can provide many hours of pleasure. Make sure the bike has lights, horn or bell, and reflectors.

When you first start cycling, it's easy to overdo it because it can seem so easy. Unless it's a gradual approach, you'll develop sore leg muscles. Some people also take a while to get used to the present design of bicycle seats.

I would suggest no more than ten to fifteen minutes of slow pedalling the first week or two. Gradually increase the time until you can achieve a continuous pace at medium speed for thirty, forty-five, and then sixty minutes or more.

There are also several well-made stationary bicycles that are built to be used in the home. There is a speedometer which measures distance and speed. One of my friends prefers this to cycling outdoors. He likes the norm of getting into his aerobic exercises in a controlled temperature environment, while listening to the radio or watching television. If you put it in the bedroom, you will see it every day and be reminded to get your exercise, no matter what.

These stationary bicycles are an ideal solution if you live in a city with heavy traffic and pollution. They are fine, although most people enjoy being outdoors in the fresh air, and like to change scenic environments whenever they can. A healthful and fun pastime can be long bicycle rides where you carry a picnic lunch. Lots of people join clubs where organized rides and other activities help provide additional motivation and enjoyment. Clubs also remind you to keep up with your exercising.

Wear comfortable clothing, good shoes, and a helmet for added safety. It's also a good idea to carry money for a phone call, a tire repair kit, tools, and an operating manual in case you run into trouble.

3. **Swimming**—If you have ready access to a pool, swimming is an ideal aerobic exercise. Once you know how to swim, you can probably gain great benefit from this exercise. People with various deficiencies and physical problems can usually swim when they can't do other exercises. Even those without the use of an arm or leg can still swim quite well.

Any of the swimming strokes can be used, but because the freestyle (or "crawl") stroke is the best known and possibly the best all-around stroke, I recommend it. Since women are generally weaker in the arm muscles than men, perhaps you can try the breast stroke. This is better for women, since it does not require the muscle strength in the arms that freestyle demands. If you aren't familiar with these strokes, or don't know how to swim well, enroll in a course with a reputable instructor. Your city, county, or neighborhood pool probably offers lessons in the summertime, and most YMCA and YWCA's offer swimming lessons year 'round.

For the first week of your aerobic swimming program, swim for only a few minutes at a time—usually one or two laps of the pool. Keep the rule about being able to speak comfortably in mind and stop if you feel out of breath, or develop pain. "Doggie paddle," tread water, or hang on to the side and kick your legs until you get your breath back before continuing. Gradually increase your work-outs until you can continue at a medium pace for thirty minutes to an hour, or more.

Swimming is considered by most medical authorities to be the most perfect of all aerobic exercises, and I share this view. Most of the muscle groups are used and there is less stress on certain body areas (like back and legs) which can occur while running or cycling.

In most areas, there are public pools with regular hours available for swimming. If it is more to your liking, look into a private swim club if they are available in your area. I've found the best time to swim is during the normal dinner hour, when most children are at home. Some pools have swim times strictly for adults.

For those who enjoy competition, there are swimming events available for all age groups, including women as well as children. Groups are divided by age, such as "Over 35," "Over 45," etc., and involve nearly all swimming strokes and distances.

As to equipment, buy a comfortable bathing suit made out of

lightweight material. For women, the "tank" style is preferred, since the straps are designed not to slip off your shoulders. Some people prefer ear and nose plugs. If you have long hair, you might prefer the type of bathing cap sold in sporting goods stores. While these don't keep you hair dry, they will keep it out of your face and free from tangles. Also, when long hair is floating around you, it tends to slow you down by creating a drag.

Moderate exposure to natural sunlight through relaxing outdoors after swimming is healthy. Since most of us spend our days indoors under artificial fluorescent lighting, sunlight can make us feel better and improve our appearance. Of course, too much exposure to the sun (to the point of burning) is harmful and can lead to skin cancer. In short doses, however, it's good for you.

4. **Walking**—For more people than ever, walking is a favorite form of exercise. It can be performed at any time, anywhere, without special equipment or facilities. In addition, it has many beneficial effects. For some, their best thinking is done while going on long enjoyable walks.

Aerobic walking, though no less enjoyable, does take a certain amount of gradual conditioning so that you may do it briskly and for sustained periods of time. Good, comfortable shoes are a must. Jogging shoes are ideal, as are low-heeled hiking boots, depending on the terrain and surface you choose. If you are not used to walking, keep your walks down to about 30 minutes the first week or so. Gradually increase until you can maintain a brisk, continuous pace for forty-five to sixty minutes.

Some may feel that the length of time needed to participate in aerobic walking is a drawback, while others find it the most enjoyable part of their day. While aerobic walking does take some time, the results (a healthier body and mind) are worth the time investment. On the matter of time, you might find as I did that you will actually seem to find more time available to you after you have been following the Total Glow program for a while. You may find that you can rise earlier and not feel as tired as you would normally, or stay up a little later and get up at your usual time. Many people do not need or require as much sleep and rest as they did previously once their overall health improves. While we all vary in the amount of sleep that we require, sometimes a poor health level causes us to sleep or rest an excessive amount of time.

Roving and Hiking

A variation of walking that you may wish to try is jogging/walking, sometimes called "roving." When roving, you jog a short distance, then walk until you catch your breath, then repeat the process. An ideal length of time to rove is one hour. Begin with a half an hour, and work up to a full hour or more. One of my clients roves daily for an hour and thoroughly enjoys it. He is in marvelous health at the age of 63, and his appearance leads people to believe that he is about 45.

Another client skips a big lunch and conducts his business meetings while taking a daily hour's walk with colleagues. He feels his best thinking is done on these jaunts. When he returns to his office, he enjoys a very light lunch—sometimes just fruit yogurt or a sandwich.

Hiking is another variation of walking that you might enjoy. A nice hike through several miles of countryside on a beautiful day is one of life's greatest pleasures. You may also enjoy a hiking club, and if you have children, you'll want to take part in the family outings. Hiking, walking, and roving are beneficial aerobic exercises for men, women, and children.

Day 3
Eating For Your Health And Happiness

Very few people realize that the business of eating can be as enjoyable as it is necessary. Although over-eating seems to be a common complaint, there are many psychological aspects involved in enjoying a good meal.

Monitoring your diet, though, and being a little bit innovative and adventurous, can net you an improved state of health and happiness with which nothing can compare.

The most prevalent complaint among over-eaters is that they can never find anything they like that isn't fattening. Taking it a step further, it is my contention that it is equally as difficult to find foods that are nutritionally worthwhile!

What is Junk Food?

Today's market is flooded with what is popularly referred to as "junk food." More appropriate, probably, would be the term "non-food." Although it is not within the scope of this book to delve into a long dissertation about the evils of non-foods since this area is receiving constant media attention, it might be apropos to say that consumption of nothing but non-food can be as bad as eating nothing at all! And it may be worse.

Human Evolution and Food

Non-food has a very large concentration of chemicals and (in many cases) additives which can accumulate in your system. In some cases these additives interfere with natural bodily processes, and in general can create all kinds of havoc in the human body. At this time the human system is simply not designed to cope with these foreign substances. Perhaps in centuries to come, humans will have evolved to the point where they can handle the extra burden.

With many of these alien elements, the long-range effects are not even known to scientists and the medical profession. Although the F.D.A. is now taking steps to investigate them and their effects on human beings, this research has been a long time coming. Still, the F.D.A. maintains that it has not been proved that these substances are harmful, and is placing the burden of proof on the nutritionists. It is my belief that they should be investigated closely, simply because it has never been proved that they are *not* harmful.

The voices of many people are being heard lately, with comments such as:

"Living on the planet Earth causes cancer."

"Living may be hazardous to your health."

"What we need are stronger, healthier laboratory rats."

The more we pay attention to known health hazards, the better off we'll be, but I must admit that at times it seems as if everything we eat or drink is potentially dangerous.

How Our Views About Food Can Hurt Us

Let us examine again some of the psychological aspects of food and eating. As a hangover from Victorian repressiveness of years ago, American people came to believe that anything pleasant or "good" was somehow evil and to be avoided at all costs in order to maintain a virtuous life. Sexual relationships fell into this category as well, and it has taken all this time to even approach being free of the hang-ups this repressiveness caused. People are finally getting to the point where they may throw off their Victorian ideals and start being human again.

Food has been likened to sex in that it is pleasant and it makes us feel good. But it seems that the same old-fashioned restrictions apply to food. How many times have you heard someone refuse a dish by saying,

"Oh, no, I shouldn't!"

When we do indulge ourselves in something really delicious, there is an underlying guilt that diminishes our enjoyment of it. There may be good reasons why some people cannot partake of certain foods, but the point is that most people feel as if they are being "bad" when they do enjoy an occassional splurge on something sweet, "fattening," or especially mouth-watering.

Unless you have a specific problem where the consumption of these kinds of things will cause you harm, there isn't really any reason why you shouldn't be able to enjoy them occasionally without the underlying guilt feelings. Especially if you are conscientious and watch what you eat most of the time, enjoying a dessert or special dish occasionally shouldn't be anything less than pleasurable.

When you have been taught (or have taught yourself) that certain foods are morally good while others are bad, this kind of psychological reinforcement becomes ingrained in your subconscious mind and it continues to work to restrain you from enjoying much of anything. The key to the Total Glow program is *moderation* in everything.

Another way in which this type of programming works is that the person blames his or her guilt on some outside authority. Whoever this authority might be (parent, teacher, sibling, spouse, clergyman) is really beside the point. It progresses to the point of near-revenge where the person over-eats to get back at the authority. In effect, they are saying, "I'll show you!" This may be rebelling against authority, but consider what you are doing to *yourself* in the meantime, and exactly whom you are hurting by this behavior.

Eventually, these types of actions become a trap for the person performing them, and we cannot seem to shake the guilt or revenge feelings. Sometimes it is carried throughout a person's lifetime, which severely limits him or her and the ability to enjoy food.

What I propose in the Total Glow program is a rational approach to diet. Every person is unique, and the design of a rigid diet plan that everyone should follow will not be attempted. This would be virtually impossible, especially since each of us has at least one favorite food, and to deprive ourselves of this one "weakness" would be setting up another authority figure against whom to rebel. We would also feel failure or guilt if we don't quite make it, and would then be saying to ourselves, "See, I knew I couldn't do it anyway."

How to Clear Up Misconceptions About Dieting

Tremendous controversy exists (and probably will exist for years to come) regarding that which is considered to be the best reducing diet. Perhaps there is no such thing, as everyone has different needs. Some people want to literally *watch* the pounds disappear, while others would prefer to feel satisfied while taking them off slowly. There is no single optimum diet for everyone, but the one that meets both your nutritional and psychological needs is the best one for you.

I would advise that you take stock of yourself, your goals, and your prerequisites before embarking upon any form of weight reduction plan. How many pounds do you need to lose? Do you simply need to shape up? How long are you willing to spend on a reducing diet plan? Are there certain foods that you simply *can't* give up?

Above all, check with your doctor, as he/she will be ultimately helpful in assisting you with the selection of the right diet for you. A physician might even be able to perform certain tests to determine your own special chemical needs, if deemed necessary.

The height/weight charts that follow are not indicative of exactly what you should weigh, but they are good general guidelines. Try to stay about five pounds on either side of it. It is important to try to avoid frequent significant changes in your weight, but minor fluctuations are normal.

MEN
Weights in Pounds (in indoor clothing)

Height (with shoes)		Small Frame	Medium Frame	Large Frame
Feet	Inches			
5	2	112-120	118-129	126-141
5	3	115-123	121-133	129-144
5	4	118-126	124-136	132-148
5	5	121-129	127-139	135-152
5	6	124-133	130-143	138-156
5	7	128-137	134-147	142-161
5	8	132-141	138-152	147-166
5	9	136-145	142-156	151-170
5	10	140-150	146-160	155-174
5	11	144-154	150-165	159-179
6	0	148-158	154-170	164-184
6	1	152-162	158-175	168-189
6	2	156-167	162-180	173-194
6	3	160-171	167-185	178-199
6	4	164-175	172-190	182-204

Your Metabolism and What It Means

Each individual on earth has a totally different biological make-up from every other individual. This can occur in the most obvious indicators—the facial features, height, bone structure, and coloring. The internal differences are even more pronounced; from the number of pancreatic cells to the variations in the blood vessel patterns in our hearts.[1] Therefore, no one can attempt to set up a reducing diet that is going to be successful for even a small percentage of the people who follow it.

As mentioned previously, a diet is not a deprivation or restriction. It is what you put into your mouth and swallow. If you are desirous of losing weight, don't use the word "diet." Think of your food intake as "what I'm trying to put *into* my body." It's not a great big splurge on eating anything, nor is your reducing diet plan the plain tea/dry toast/cottage cheese misery of years ago. Your diet is what you eat. If you want to lose weight, that is something else entirely.

Do you ever hear the statement, "The person who lives next door to me can eat anything she wants and never gains a pound! If I even get close enough to *smell* something, I gain weight!"? Somebody then probably put the person down and made them feel guilty by saying some-

WOMEN
Weights in Pounds (in indoor clothing)

Height (with shoes)		Small Frame	Medium Frame	Large Frame
Feet	Inches			
4	10	92- 98	96-107	104-119
4	11	94-101	98-110	106-122
5	0	96-104	101-113	109-125
5	1	99-107	104-116	112-128
5	2	102-110	107-119	115-131
5	3	105-113	110-122	118-134
5	4	108-116	113-126	121-138
5	5	111-119	116-130	125-142
5	6	114-123	120-135	129-146
5	7	118-127	124-139	133-150
5	8	122-131	128-143	137-154
5	9	126-135	132-147	141-158
5	10	130-140	136-151	145-163
5	11	134-144	140-155	149-168
6	0	138-148	144-159	153-173

---

[1] Roger J. Williams, Ph.D., *You Are Extraordinary* (New York: Pyramid Publications, 1967).

Normal Height—Weight, Ages ½ to 21 Years

AGE	MALE		FEMALE	
Years	Height Inches	Weight Pounds	Height Inches	Weight Pounds
½	26	17	26	16
1	29	21	29	20
2	33	26	33	25
3	36	31	36	30
4	39	35	39	34
5	42	38	41	37
6	45	43	44	43
7	47	50	47	47
8	49	55	49	54
9	51	61	51	60
10	53	67	53	67
11	55	75	55	74
12	57	81	57	82
13	59	90	60	94
14	62	103	62	105
15	64	112	63	112
16	66	126	64	117
17	67	133	64	122
18	68	138	65	124
19	69	138	65	126
20	69	139	65	126

thing like, "Well, that's impossible. You must be cheating on your diet." They may know that they have not been eating that much and certainly not doing any "cheating," yet they still have trouble losing weight.

It isn't surprising that this happens. Just as we all do different jobs, have different likes and dislikes, and enjoy different things, so it is that we are all uniquely individual in the ways in which our bodies metabolize the food that we consume. There are many different types of metabolism in humans, and it often changes throughout the years. If you have always been extra-thin, you may think that you are exempt from the problem of obesity forever, but in most cases, this isn't true.[2]

The body stops growing "up" at about the age of twenty-five or thirty and tends to slow down somewhat. It is this age when those super-thin people begin to notice the pounds accumulating. They blame it on their jobs where they're sitting all day, or having a baby, or any number of things that they claim are beyond their control. The simple truth is that their metabolism has changed. It has slowed down, and these people will have to be careful about what they eat for the rest of their lives, just like the rest of us.

Perhaps it is hardest on these people to re-adjust themselves to watching their weight. They have fond memories of gleefully bingeing on milkshakes, pizzas, candy, soft drinks, and sweets, and never gaining an ounce. These people have to dramatically change their thinking or, sadly, they will eventually become overweight and will suffer from all the crippling diseases that go along with it.

If you are one of those people who have always had to watch your weight, chances are that your metabolism is such that your body has difficulty converting starches and sugars into energy. This is not an uncommon condition. Your carbohydrates are turning into fat instead of being converted to glucose and being burned up. Your body starts storing the fat in unbecoming places.

The usual weight reducing plan contains approximately fifty percent carbohydrates. If your metabolism is such that you cannot effectively assimilate carbohydrates, this is obviously not going to do you much good. If you have followed this type of reducing diet plan strictly for more than a year and have not been able to realize any appreciable, permanent weight loss, it would be recommended that you have a frank discussion with your doctor.

Ask about increasing the amount of protein and fat in your diet plan and reducing carbohydrate intake. If you are one of those people who seems to gain weight just by smelling something fattening, it is entirely possible that this is exactly what's happening! At this point in your life, you have a different metabolic rate than the super-thin people. The best thing you can do for yourself is to speak with your physician and try to get back in touch with your body. Listen to what it trys to tell you when you eat something.

---

[2]William D. Kelly, M.D., *The Various Metabolic Types* (Washington, D.C.: lecture, The Nutritional Academy, January, 1978).

How to Listen to Your Body

If you eat something very sweet, do you feel ready to go scale the Empire State Building, or do you feel slightly dizzy and disoriented? How often does your body tell you that it craves something like fish or spinach? Have you ever had an inexplicable desire for a good steak-and-potatoes meal? Do you sometimes pass up dessert just so you'll have room enough for some more of that delicious salad?

These are all examples of the ways in which your body can tell you what it needs, and how it reacts to what you feed it. Listen. You'll be surprised.

Try not to be too jealous of the super-thins, who can gorge themselves on food and not gain weight. Most of them will be much worse off than you are in a few years, and the adjustment will be many times more difficult. Start keeping a close eye on what you are eating and how you feel afterwards.

Does food make you sleepy? Do you get an upset stomach after combining certain kinds of foods? What happens when you don't drink anything with your meal? If you stopped eating sugar for a week, how would you feel on the seventh day? Watch to see exactly what happens when you do gain a few pounds. Where does it go? Does it show up on the scales, in the mirror, or is it merely a tight, bloated feeling? *When* do you gain weight, and when do you lose it?

On the following pages, I have included charts whereby you can conveniently keep track of everything you eat for a week. Record what you ate, when, and how you felt afterwards. Increased awareness of our diets and our emotions is crucial to understanding ourselves and our needs.

This chart is not a confessional-type exercise, and you don't have to think of it as such. It will be interesting to see what your eating habits are later, and to try to discern how different foods affect you. There are certain foods to which you might be allergic, that effect you in different ways at different times of day. Also, your tolerance levels change. For example, drinking fruit juice first thing in the morning might cause some people to have indigestion, while juice is tolerated much better in the afternoon and evening. If you skip a meal, try to pay attention to how you feel.

One person reported to me her discovery of the effects of coffee. She found one morning that she was particularly jittery and seemed to be overly anxious about a few random, insignificant things. Looking back to what she had ingested that morning, she discovered that she'd had several cups of strong coffee—much more than normal for her. Trying an experiment, she waited a few days, then drank a large amount of coffee. The mildly irrational fears and nervousness returned. Try to be as aware of your body as this person was.

"WHAT I EAT"

First Day: List everything that you put into your mouth (including coffee, gum, candy, or other snacks)

Food

Breakfast: Snack/Coffee Break:

_____   _____

_____   _____

_____   _____

Lunch: Snack/Coffee Break:

_____   _____

_____   _____

_____   _____

Dinner: Snack:

_____   _____

_____   _____

_____   _____

Second Day:

Breakfast: Snack/Coffee Break:

_____   _____

_____   _____

_____   _____

Lunch: Snack/Coffee Break:

_____   _____

_____   _____

_____   _____

Dinner: Snack:

_____   _____

_____   _____

_____   _____

Third Day:

Breakfast: Snack/Coffee Break:

_____   _____

_____   _____

_____   _____

Lunch: Snack/Coffee Break:

_____   _____

_____   _____

_____   _____

Dinner: Snack:

_____   _____

_____   _____

_____   _____

Fourth Day:

Breakfast: Snack/Coffee Break:

_____   _____

_____   _____

_____   _____

Lunch: Snack/Coffee Break:

_____   _____

_____   _____

_____   _____

Dinner: _____

Snack: _____

Fifth Day:

Breakfast: _____

Snack/Coffee Break: _____

Lunch: _____

Snack/Coffee Break: _____

Dinner: _____

Snack: _____

Day 3 Eating For Your Health And Happiness

What do your eating habits tell you? Are you satisfied that they are healthy, or, like most of us, did the amount or quality of your diet surprise you? Oftentimes, we are never really aware of what we're eating, and keeping track of it can have eye-opening results.

Here are some more questions to help you become more aware of your diet:

Diet Awareness Questionnaire

1. Describe the lunch most of your fellow workers or friends eat each day: _____

_____

_____

2. List what your children (or relatives' and friends' children) eat for breakfast each day: _____

_____

_____

3. Read the labels on the above products. Are there any ingredients you may be confused about? If so, list them: _____

_____

_____

_____

106 Total Glow

4. Five of the easiest ways I can help my children get off non-nutritious junk foods are:
   1.

   2.

   3.

   4.

   5.

5. Some of the hardest things for them to avoid will be: _____

_____

_____

_____

6. Some of the ways I can help my family, especially the children, avoid embarrassment resulting from peer pressure about changing their eating habits would be: _____

_____

_____

_____

7. Whether I am adult or teenager, some of the best ways to avoid embarrassment about my new health program are: _____

_____

_____

_____

Learn to carry a little notebook with you to keep track of your eating habits on a continuing basis. Don't worry if you forget to list a few meals or snacks, simply list what you are eating next time. Remember that one of our biggest hindrances when starting anything new is giving up because we "fall off" for a time. It takes time to change and learn new habits, and it will help you to remember that no person ever did it without a few regressions and mistakes.

Once you have some concrete answers to the kinds of questions I asked about food and how it makes you feel, you will be able to intelligently formulate your own weight reduction plan. Throw out all your diet books, stop taking everyone else's advice about favorite weight reducing diets, and do some hard thinking about yourself. Plan a weight reduction effort for *your* body, that is as unique as you are.

If salt makes you bloat with water, cut out the salt. If sugar makes you feel lethargic, don't eat it. Contrary to popular opinion, all of us can live without *any* refined sugar in our diets. (If this wasn't so, we wouldn't have very many diabetic people around who live virtually without sugar.) If red meat makes your stomach ache or gives you indigestion, cut down on it. Oriental people live almost exclusively on fish and vegetables. There is hardly anything in the standard American diet that some healthy people somewhere in the world don't live entirely without.

Try to break out of the conditioning that is leading you into unhealthy eating habits. Just because you've been eating certain kinds of foods all your life doesn't mean that they are necessarily good for you.

You are unique. You are extraordinary, as the saying goes. You are the best thing you've got. Give yourself the most margin possible to lead the healthiest and happiest of lives. You deserve it.

Regardless of the areas of controversy, a healthy body that is well-nourished is going to be better able to fight off diseases and illnesses than a worn-out, over-stressed one. A fatigued and distressed body does not necessarily come from aging, as is commonly believed, but from the way in which it is cared for. Certain degenerative processes are inevitable and cannot be averted, but many of the so-called "aches and pains" of growing older can be eliminated through proper care and nutrition.

There isn't any quick pill, easy weight reduction plan, or magical formula that can rejuvenate all the millions of cells comprising all the different organs in your body. This kind of effort takes time, patience, and loving care. You may be doing yourself the biggest favor possible by viewing your self-care effort as an interesting and enjoyable endeavor. Think of it as a hobby; something into which you will be putting a great deal of time and effort, but one in which the return investment will be hundred-fold.

In learning to prepare your own healthful meals, you'll find that cooking and working in the kitchen is a highly creative and relaxing endeavor. Not many men have had the opportunity of exploring the thrill of cooking and turning out a really excellent meal. Cooking carries with it many of the things that men typically enjoy: working with their hands, experimentation, imagination, and (most of all) testing the grand results.

Most men who have tried their hands in the kitchen have become marvelously imaginative cooks. If you think of it, the majority of the world's great chefs have been men. Many of the standard American favorites were also created by men who started "fooling around" in their wives' kitchens. The founder of the world's healthiest ice cream, Haagen Daaz, is an example of this.

So it would seem that men are particularly adept at cooking, and all are encouraged to give it a try. The recipes included in the Total Glow program are easy to prepare and can be modified to suit most any taste or creative inclination.

As you look through the recipes, several important points should be kept in mind. These are guidelines presented to facilitate your understanding of the basic concepts of the program and healthier eating:

Steps to Healthier Eating

1. Try to take positive control of your diet. For a great many people, the food is controlling them, not the other way around. Do some reading. Investigate. Be adventurous. Accept the responsibility for what you eat, and decide that you are going to improve in this area.

2. Increase the amount of fresh and raw foods in your diet. Try to achieve a ratio of sixty percent raw to forty percent cooked. The raw foods have retained their nutrients and are much more valuable. You might get into this new habit slowly by eating a salad with lunch and dinner, and enjoying more fresh fruits for breakfast and desserts. This will also increase the fiber in your diet.

3. Decrease the amount of preservatives and additives in all your food through intelligent shopping and trips to health food stores.

4. Avoid frequent use of overly processed foods unless you know for a fact that they are basically free of additives and harm-

ful chemicals. It's on the label.

5. Use as many natural foods and products as you can. Start substituting natural sugars for refined, as you gradually cut down on the amount of sugar in your diet entirely.

6. Use natural, cold-pressed oils (such as sesame and olive, which are most resistant to rancidity). Avoid all hard animal fats that will not melt at room temperature, and those oils that are artificially processed.

7. Make your own fresh healthy foods using the recipes included in the Total Glow program. Remember not to cook or heat any vegetable oil over 250° as it releases carcinogenic agents at that temperature and above.[3]

8. Check your water supply. The amount of chlorine added to counteract other pollutants in many areas has reached alarming levels. If necessary, switch to distilled water and add mineral supplements to your diet. Your health food proprietor should be able to help you in this respect. In terms of having your water supply tested, the Environmental Protection Agency is the one to contact, or there are usually private companies for this service. (Incidentally, the E.P.A. checked our water supply several times to make sure the results were accurate—they couldn't believe it was as bad as it was! We are now using distilled water exclusively for drinking and cooking.)

9. Read all labels carefully. Make sure you are buying only those items free of preservatives, additives, nitrates and nitrites, colorings, and artificial substances. If you don't feel as if you can completely eliminate these things from your diet, try to use them in moderation. Even in a health food store, be certain to read labels and ask about the products. Many unhealthy substances infiltrate some health food stores.

10. Develop a healthful consciousness whereby you will be able to adapt these guidelines to your life and follow them without too great an effort.

11. Look for the following items in your health food store, and try to convince your grocer to stock them in the supermarket:

A. *Juices*—an abundance of fresh juices are available in the refrigerated section. These are free from additives, preservatives, and artificial coloring. I usually dilute natural fruit and vegetable juices with water, as they are more potent tast-

---

[3] Airola, Paavo, Ph. D., N. D. — lecture, Washington, D. C., April, 1978

ing. Squeeze your own juice as often as possible.

B. *Bread*—why not develop a talent for baking your own bread? There are many new brands appearing on the shelves, however, that contain various health-promoting grains that are free from preservatives. Use whole grain breads and check to be sure that whole wheat is fresh, since it goes rancid rapidly. Stick with rye and unbleached types of bread, or obtain fresh whole wheat for baking.

C. *Seasonings*—keep various types of organic seasonings (such as kelp, parakelp, tamari soy sauce, sea salt, and herbs) on hand and use them as often as you like. With time, you will learn the proper amount for your taste. Herbs, especially, will cut down on the amount of salt you feel you need. Sea salt is healthier than table salt because it contains essential minerals that have been removed from table salt.

D. *Soup bases/Stocks*—when fresh stock is not available, look for natural, organic stocks such as onion, vegetable, beef, and chicken.

E. *Crackers and "munchies"*—many "100% Natural" snacks are appearing on the market. *Read* the labels to make sure, and buy these instead of junk food. Make your own snacks from Total Glow recipes.

F. *Jams/Jellies*—even the major food manufacturers are introducing lines of natural jams, jellies, preserves, and marmalades, but these still have refined sugar. Also available in health food stores are many flavors of natural concentrated sweeteners in fruits such as cherry, cranberry, and apricot. These are great added to your homemade cereal, yogurt shakes, and other dishes that could use a flavor or sweetener.

G. *Pasta*—there are many types of non-preservative, low-calorie pasta available which are made from bases such as artichoke and spinach. Use these pastas in your spaghetti, lasagna, linguini, and other noodle dishes for a different and exciting taste.

H. *Flour*—grocery stores are now stocking unbleached flours in quantity. Another good substitute is arrowroot, which is a ground root, and it stores well at room temperature. Arrowroot is probably the least processed of any available flour, and least likely to become rancid and carcinogenic.

I. *Chocolate*—carob, which is rich in calcium, magnesium, iron, potassium, and other vitamins and minerals is a great substitute for chocolate. Chocolate consumes calcium, and too much of it could be a bad thing. Carob produces a beneficial alkaline reaction in your system which combats the calcium removal of chocolate. Add carob to milkshakes and other recipes calling for chocolate and cocoa. Carob comes in sweetened or unsweetened form.

J. *Sugar*—In general, the natural sweeteners are best. In moderation, the artificial sweeteners can be substituted when there is over-consumption of refined sugar in your diet. Until the issue of saccharin is finally resolved, I would recommend that while using it, eliminate it from your diet for a full week every three weeks so that your body can be totally free of it. This way, it won't build up in your system. Try to use the fruit sweeteners already mentioned whenever you can, but don't rush yourself into kicking a sugar habit. When your body is saturated with refined sugar, you might feel shaky, nervous, and irritable if you suddenly stop ingesting it. It takes time to rid yourself of the accumulated refined sugar in your system.

K. *Mayonnaise*—Instructions for making your own completely natural mayonnaise are included in the recipe section, or you can obtain non-preservative mayonnaise in a health food store made with safflower or sesame oil.

L. *Raw nuts and grains*—Nothing is more delicious than roasting your own peanuts, cashews, almonds, or chestnuts. When buying nuts in the store, avoid the overly salted and processed brands. Raw nuts are readily available in health food stores and are a delicious treat when they are soaked overnight in fruit juice or tamari soy sauce. Grains are perhaps one of the single most healthful foods available.

M. *Dried fruits*—These contain no additives or preservatives, and are great when mixed with raw nuts and seeds for a snack. Drying foods is one of the best ways of preserving them, as they lose far fewer nutrients than through freezing or canning.

N. *Peas/Lentils/Beans*—Often it is best to buy the dried type and make your own rather than using the canned variety. Again, recipes are included in the following sections. Legumes are a good source of protein and fiber.

O. *Grain Cereals*—Making your own cereal is a great project and quite often you will discover that yours is far superior to the processed kind. Again, they are high in protein and fiber. See the recipes in the following sections.

P. *Salad Dressings*—There are many of these mixes available that are natural and without preservatives, in flavors ranging from bleu cheese to Caesar. They make delicious dressings as well as dips for snacks.

Q. *Herbs*—Consider growing your own herbs or buy them through the health food store.

R. *Relishes/Pickles/Condiments*—These, too, are available in natural form without preservatives, and are quite good. You might even try making your own using honey instead of sugar, and fresh herbs and spices.

S. *Meats/Poultry/Fish*—Look for stores carrying products derived from animals raised without chemicals or drugs. Always check for freshness and try to determine (in the case of fish and shellfish) where they were caught. Generally, the farther out from shoreline, the less contaminated they will be.

T. *Baking Powder*—Use cellulow sodium baking powder. The problem with sodium bicarbonate (common baking powder) is that it tends to inactivate the vitamins in your food. Substitute the potassium bicarbonate baking powder where you normally use ordinary baking soda.

U. *Pepper*—Black pepper can be toxic and hard for the kidneys to handle. Substitute cayenne pepper or dried ground papaya seeds.

V. *Eggs*—I highly recommend the use of fertile eggs. These come from chickens with roosters around them, and can be purchased in health food stores or from some farms. Fertile hens have been raised in a natural environment and have not been fed additives, preservatives, and chemicals or foods to fatten them quickly. When using raw eggs in a recipe, run very hot tap water over the egg shell before cracking. This destroys an enzyme within the membrane of the egg which can inhibit some of the B vitamins.

W. *Bee Pollen*—Studies have shown that bee pollen helps to combat viruses for which antibiotics, antihistamines, and other drugs do not seem to help.

How To Get More Nutrients From The Food You Eat

1. Eat whole grains daily or at least five times a week. If you have a seed mill, you can buy the whole grains and crack them yourself. Use it in preparing your own cereals, sprinkle some on salads, on top of yogurt, and in yogurt shakes.

2. Steam your vegetables with only one or two tablespoons of water. Do not overcook vegetables as they are very delicate and lose their nutrients very easily. Eat them crunchy. Up to 50% more vitamin loss occurs when you add more water in cooking.

3. Save the left-over liquid from steaming vegetables. Keep it frozen and substitute it for water in soups, stocks, and other vegetable recipes.

4. Always eat the skins on vegetables and fruits unless they are waxy or artificial in appearance. The center core of vegetables like cucumbers and cabbage are also very nutritious.

5. Use tightly fitting lids when steaming vegetables so that the nutrients do not escape.

6. A small pressure cooker is a time saver and insures protection of nutrients, as you need very little water.

7. Cut and slice vegetables as close to the time of using them as possible. Tear lettuce-type vegetables rather than cutting. Add salad dressings just before eating.

8. Do not wash vegetables until ready to use. Nutrients leave the produce and go down the drain with the water. If you soak vegetables, retain the water as in #3 above.

9. After shopping, refrigerate your green vegetables as soon as possible. If you leave them in the car to do other errands, they lose vitamins A and C.

10. Peppers, eggplants, and cucumber are best stored in paper bags or in crisper without wrapping, as plastic bags will make them soggy. Keeping leafy greens in plastic bags will help them retain their crispness.

11. Cutting, chopping, and crushing vegetables increases their loss of the water-soluble vitamins since you are increasing the surface area

and freeing enzymes that cause the loss of water-soluble vitamins.

12. Defrost meats in the refrigerator rather than under water or at room temperature.

13. Do not salt meat before or during cooking. Salt extracts all the juices, making the meat dry.

14. Don't overcook fish. It is quite surprising how little time it takes to cook fresh fish. Cook only until flesh is white and flakey—any more than that and you are killing the nutrients.

15. Serve leftover meats as cold slices or in salads. Reheating destroys more Vitamin B.

16. Toast bread only lightly since the heating removes nutrients.

A Critical Look At Sugar
Some Startling Facts You Probably Didn't Know

Do you have any of the following symptoms frequently?

irritability	muscle cramps
anxiety	blurry vision
exhaustion	impotence
nervousness	sexual wantonness
dizziness	illusion of smothering
light headedness	feelings of impending disaster
confusion	fears and phobias
trembling	rapid heart beat
tingling in extremities	drowsiness
increased anxiety	restlessness
insomnia	headaches
sudden skin disorders	adult acne

If you suffer from one or more of these symptoms regularly, and your doctor has not been able to attribute them to some other ailment, chances are that you have been ingesting too much refined sugar. Does that surprise you?

This isn't to say that you gorge yourself on sweets or desserts, or that you are a fiend with the sugar bowl. It simply means that there is so much hidden sugar in the normal American diet that you could be overdosing yourself and not even know it!

Most people will admit it when they have become addicted to something like coffee or cigarettes, but few are even aware that they could possibly be addicted to sugar.

Refined sugar is included in almost every product on supermarket shelves. For an eye-opening and sometimes shocking account of the diseases and malaise refined sugar has wrecked upon the people of the world, read *Sugar Blues* by William Dufty. To illustrate a few examples by this author, he states that it has been historically documented that scurvvy, beriberi, and pelagra are the direct result of the refining processes of sugar, rice, and flour. He also states that he recovered from undiagnosed (and therefore untreated) ailments and diseases when he kicked his sugar habit of many years.[4]

The more refined sugar that you ingest ($C_{12}H_{22}O_{11}$), the more your pancreas and liver have to work to handle it. If you wake up in the morning and have a breakfast that largely consists of sugar, you will probably get off to an energetic start. But you will soon develop cravings, then take a coffee and donut break, adding more sugar. Throughout the day, you will be feeling up and down, all depending upon the amount of refined sugar you have ingested.

When your system is overloaded with sugar, the pancreas works harder to produce more insulin. You then begin to feel nervous, cranky, and perhaps even nauseated. You eat more sugar, in one form or another, and your pancreas over-reacts once again, producing more insulin and resulting in the nervousness or, in many people, depression, all over again. See the merry-go-'round effect?

When you don't overload your system with refined sugar, your organs can maintain an even level of insulin. Your emotions, not to mention your physical health, will be on a much more even keel.

To give you an example of how much hidden sugar (refined sugar that is disguised in processed foods and packaging) the average person ingests, the magazine *"Let's Live"* recently reported 110 pounds per year per person. This is more than *forty tablespoons* daily per person!!

The need for vitamins and minerals increases with sugar intake. Since refined sugar has been stripped of all its nutritional content, it cannot be turned into energy without certain vitamins, especially the B_1 thiamine group.

Natural sugars that are found in fruits, vegetables, grains, and honey partially make up for the deficiency created by refined sugar, since the B vitamins have not been removed. Beware, however, of certain forms of "raw sugar" being sold in many stores. On further investigation, it was found to be refined sugar to which brown food coloring had been added to make it appear unrefined. Ask! Read labels!

---

[4]William Dufty, *Sugar Blues* (New York: Warner Books, Inc., 1975).

Another way that the sugar is hidden is through the labeling of products containing it. The food industry has lumped sugar with all other carbohydrates. A breakfast cereal with a label indicating twenty-two grams of carbohydrate per cup does indeed have twenty-two grams of carbohydrate. But that carbohydrate, or at least a major portion of it, may be in the form of refined sugar. To get a better idea of exactly how much of the carbohydrate count is actually sugar in any product, read the label and the ingredients listed. Manufacturers must list the ingredients in descending order, so if sugar is listed first or appears within the first four ingredients, you can make a safe bet that the carbohydrate count is almost entirely refined sugar.

Also watch out for different names for sugar. Usually if the word has "-ose" on the end of it, as in sucrose or frutose, it's sugar. Corn syrup is also refined sugar.

Consumer groups are now working to tighten up the food labeling laws so that carbohydrates are broken down into refined sugars, chemical sugars, and natural carbohydrates like grains and flours.

Did you know that an average serving of cherry pie has approximately fourteen tablespoons of refined sugar, and if you top if off with ice cream, that adds another five tablespoons? Or that one serving of chocolate cake with icing has fifteen tablespoons of refined sugar in it? You can find it in the most alarming places—ketchup, salad dressings, cigarettes (yes, cigarettes), table salt, tomato soup, clam chowder, spaghetti sauce, canned vegetables—and this isn't to mention the obvious things like ice cream, breakfast cereals, commercial yogurt, canned fruit, and soft drinks.

It would be wise to develop your own sugar alarm system where you can detect the most minute quantities of refined sugar. As you free yourself from the habit, your taste buds will be able to pick it up. Until the labeling laws made it somewhat clearer, though still not adequate, you can imagine the problems diabetics had with canned, frozen, and processed foods. They had no idea how much refined sugar was getting into their diets, and this most assuredly made control of the disease difficult. Perhaps this is one reason why so many diabetics are termed "brittle diabetics" meaning that they are totally unable to control the level of sugar in their blood. Once they are able to monitor the amount of sugar they are actually ingesting by getting away from processed foods, the "brittle" and uncontrollable element disappears.

Sugar Awareness Chart

"How Sweet? Here's the Percentage of Sugar Consumer's Union Found in 24 Common Foods.
Cremora — 59%
Coffeemate — 65.4%
Coca Cola — 8.8%
Skippy Peanut Butter — 9.2%
Del Monte Whole Kernel Corn — 10.7%
Libbys Peach Halves (Canned) — 17.9%
Dannon Blueberry Lowfat Yogurt — 13.7%
Quaker 100% Natural Cereal — 23.9%
Wylers Beef Flavor Bouillon Cubes — 14.8%
Hamburger Helper — 23%
Ragu Spaghetti Sauce — 6.2%
Cool Whip (large size) — 21%
Ritz Crackers — 11.8%
Wishbone Italian Dressing — 7.3%
Wishbone Sweet and Spicy French Dressing — 23%
Wishbone Russian Dressing — 30.2%
Jell-o Cherry Flavored Gelatin — 82.6%
Sara Lee Chocolate Cake — 35.9%
Sealtest Ice Cream Parlor Ice Cream — 21.4%
Heinz Tomato Ketchup — 28.9%
Shake 'n Bake (Italian Flavor) — 14.7%
Shake 'n Bake (Original Flavor) — 17.4%
Shake 'n Bake (Chicken) — 50.9%
Kellogg's Sugar Frosted Flakes — 39%
Kellogg's Apple Jacks—57%"

This chart was derived from *Consumer Reports,* March 1978, pp. 136–141.

A Clearer Understanding of Salt

When mention is made of salt, we are essentially speaking about sodium. The human organism needs approximately one half a gram of salt per day, yet most people consume twenty times that much. In fact, a 2,000 mg. (two grams) salt diet is considered to be a "low salt" diet, even when the body only needs about 500 mg. This shows you how much we are out of touch in this whole area.

Many cultures add salt to their food because so much of the original flavor is lost in cooking and processing. Salt, like sugar, gives back some of the taste. Eventually, people become addicted to salty foods; and most often the addiction started in infancy when canned baby foods were salted to please the taste of the mother.

Often, the only time a person will voluntarily cut down on salt intake is when a doctor delivers an ultimatum. The reasons for reducing consumption of salt are many, but two major ones are that it causes you to retain fluids and that it plays a major role in high blood pressure and subsequent heart disease.

The famous nutrition magazine *"Prevention"* has stated that they will no longer list salt as an ingredient in their recipes due to the overwhelming evidence that it leads to hypertension. Perhaps this is a word to the wise.

Herbs are good substitutes for salt, and you might consider trying some salt substitutes to use intermittently with your sea salt and herbal blends. It is always easier to wean yourself from a bad habit *before* it becomes a "do or die" situation and you get the warning from your doctor.

Remember, though, that sea salt still has sodium (Na) in it. The sodium content of kelp is about 18% compared to sea salt which is 75% sodium. Brands such as "Lite Salt" are available at supermarkets and contain about 50% potassium and 50% sodium. Many people find these to be good substitutes to help reduce their intake of salt.[5]

Try your best to begin eliminating table salt from your diet. Eating fresh produce will help, as will the substitution of herbs, tamari, garlic, and natural seasonings. Eventually, you will begin to realize the many wonderful tastes of foods that had previously been masked with salt.

When discussing the unit of measurement, the milligram is used primarily. This is a metric unit of measure and is commonly used in all nutritional and medical articles. It also appears on the labels of some products. For that reason, it is important to understand it. The abbreviation of milligram is "mg." Basically, this is how much a mg. is:

1000 mg.=1 gram
½ teaspoon=1000 mg.
¼ teaspoon=500 mg.

We can do with 500 mg. or ¼ teaspoon of salt daily, or less. If you purchased only salt-free canned and frozen goods and never ate in restaurants, it would still be difficult to avoid taking in 100 to 500 mg. of salt per day.

---

[5]J. I. Rodale and Staff, *The Complete Book of Minerals for Health* (Emmaus, Pennsylvania: Rodale Books, Inc., 1976).

I don't add any salt to my cooking and buy only canned products that are not salted. Unless you are on a special diet recommended by a physician, there isn't any special reason to use salt. It is added only because it gives tastes back to the food that was lost during the processing.

If you do use salt, it's best to switch to sea salt, since it contains the trace minerals that are removed from table salt.

Most of us have no idea how much salt we are really ingesting per day. To give you a more concrete idea of the salt content of some common foods, I have prepared the chart that follows.

Salt Awareness Chart

	(Na) Sodium	Calories
*Canadian Bacon, 1 oz.	442 mg.	60
*Beef Pot Pie (commercial 7½ oz. serving)	791 mg.	415
*Beef Vegetable Stew (canned, 1 cup)	1007 mg.	194
*Homemade Beef Vegetable Stew (1 cup)	91 mg.	194
*Cake—white (1 sm. piece, unfrosted)	195 mg.	250
*Chicken Chow Mein (canned, 1 cup, no noodles)	725 mg.	95
*Corned Beef Hash (canned, 3 oz. serving)	459 mg.	154
*Soups (canned, diluted with water):		
Beef Bouillon Broth (1 cup)	784 mg.	30
Beef Noodle (1 cup)	955 mg.	70
Cream of Mushroom (1 cup)	827 mg.	135
Tomato (1 cup)	970 mg.	90
*Tomatoes:		
Raw, 1 medium	5 mg.	35
Canned, ½ cup	157 mg.	25
Pureed, 1 cup	994 mg.	97
Juice, ½ cup (canned)	242 mg.	23
Catsup, 1 tablespoon	177 mg.	15
*Apple, 1 medium	1 mg.	60
*Asparagus, 6 stalks:		
Fresh or cooked	1 mg.	18
Canned	227 mg.	20
*Banana, 1 medium	1 mg.	88
*Barley, cooked, 1 cup	1 mg.	98
*Bean sprouts, raw, 1 cup	5 mg.	30
*½ teaspoon table salt	500 mg.	

You can see how easily your salt intake becomes exceptionally high, almost without your being aware of it. Compare the content of salt in raw and fresh food to their canned/processed counterparts.

Additives and Preservatives in Your Life: Do They Belong There?

I believe our culture has been brainwashed to some extent into believing that certain preservatives in our foods are beneficial. People tend to believe that if the preservatives are not there, something terrible could happen to us; that we would suffer food poisoning or some such calamity might befall us.

The addition of *some* preservatives in *certain types* of food may be important, especially the canned varieties when prolonged shelf life is necessary. For instance, we would certainly want to preserve food that was sheltered in case of a national disaster. But at the same time, it is important to begin thinking about some of the disadvantages of preservatives in nearly all of the foods that we eat. It is my contention that all these chemical preservatives simply are *not* essential, nor are they healthy.

There seems to be a national preoccupation with adding chemicals to foods that have no real need of them. Perhaps this stems from the days before adequate refrigeration was available. When the chemists finally discovered a way to retard food spoilage through artificial additives, the discovery was hailed as a life-saving one. Didn't anyone stop to think, though, that the refrigerator had been invented in the meantime and that the problem leading to the solution no longer existed?

Why is it that Americans believe they need preservatives in food that is normally eaten soon after it is purchased? Why are there preservatives in bread, cakes, cookies, cereals, crackers, and, most incomprehensibly, in frozen foods? Somehow, people have let themselves be duped into believing that all the chemicals were necessary.

A friend once asked in alarm, "How could I eat bread that doesn't have preservatives?" The answer is simple. If you, your mother, or your grandmother ever made homemade bread, you ate bread without preservatives. Chances are it was the most delicious bread you'd ever eaten, too. Might it be that part of the great attraction and taste of homemade bread comes from the fact that all the ingredients are as natural and fresh as they can be?

Granted, many white breads that people make in their homes today are made with refined sugar and bleached white flour, but the fact remains that homemade bread is virtually free from odd-sounding chemical names that you can't pronounce. Maybe that's what makes it so good.

It is a fact of life that some food spoils. Even food with preservatives in it spoils if you leave it for too long in the refrigerator. Bread that you buy in stores will develop mold if you leave it on the counter too long. If you are concerned about molds on preservative-free bread, store it in the freezer and simply remove the number of slices you need at the time. Any food is going to spoil after a time, whether it has preservatives in it or not. So why eat chemicals that you can't even pronounce?

BHT/BHA

Substantial research simply does not exist to establish the safety of such things as BHT and BHA. These initials stand for yard-long, multisyllabled words that only the scientist who dreamed them up could love. An article in the Australian Medical Journal reported that the administration of BHT to pregnant mice had resulted in the birth of fifteen percent of the young without eyesight. Both the British and German governments have considered banning the use of this preservative. The German government made one exception only; that it be allowed in emergency rations for use by the armed forces where a long-term shelf life is necessary.

BHT is banned in Romania and Sweden, yet in the United States it continues to appear in thousands of American foods, such as breakfast cereals, breads, chewing gum, and salad oils, to mention only a few of the wide range of choices.

BHT was, in fact, used to preserve color in motion pictures! In spite of these bans, the U.S. continues to allow its use as an antioxidant to preserve foods. Yet the F.D.A. has not released any information to guarantee its safety.[6] Foods have their own natural anti-oxidents which are destroyed in high temperature processing.

---

[6]Carlton Fredericks, *Look Younger, Feel Healthier* (New York: Grosset and Dunlap, 1977).

Some Substances Found In An Ordinary Carton Of Ice Cream

Some of the other substances that are added to food are listed below, as found in an ordinary carton of ice cream:
- Diethyl Glucol—*used as an emulsifier. It is a cheap chemical which is also used in anti-freeze and paint removers.*
- Formic Acid—*a synthetic flavoring used to imitate fruit flavors. It produces violet burns and is used to de-hair animal hides.*
- Butraldehyde—*is used in nut-flavored ice cream. It is also used in rubber cement.*
- Benzaldehyde—*is used in making artifical oil of almond, coconut, apricot, and other fruit flavors. It can cause central nervous system depression and convulsions, and is potentially fatal.*
- Amyl Acetate—*is used as an imitation banana flavoring. It is also used as an oil paint solvent.*
- Piperonal—*is used in place of vanilla. It is also used in perfumes and as a lice-killer.*

A common argument made by people who are reluctant to accept the natural way is that all food is essentially chemical, and additives are simply more of the same. The body cannot tell the difference. This is a specious argument at its worst. While it is quite true that all foods are basically chemical in nature, the fact remains that the human body has had centuries to evolve so that it can absorb, digest, and assimilate all that is available on earth in natural form for consumption. It has not been until the last fifty years or so that artificial additives have been added to our food supply. These things overload, short-circuit, and poison the body, interferring with its attempts to extract the essential nutrients from whole, natural foods.

The Organs of Detoxification

The primary organs which serve to un-poison or detoxify the food we eat are the liver, kidneys, lungs, skin, and colon (large intestine). These seem to be the main organs that have in past years been most susceptible to failure, break-down, malfunction, and disease.

Perhaps it might be possible that in the coming years the human body will evolve so that it may cope with all the toxins and interference we are putting into it, but each person will be healthier TODAY if we clean out our systems and refrain from polluting ourselves further with substances that we know nothing about.

What Medical Tests Cannot Tell You

As modern medicine exists today, it is extremely difficult to diagnose a problem until it makes itself readily apparent. Surely you have heard of the number of cases of people who, having been tested and having received a clean bill of health from their physicians only hours or days before, suddenly drop dead of heart attacks. All the blood tests, urinalyses, mechanical and chemical tests in the world will not tell you a thing until something is *really* wrong. Usually, when a problem does manifest itself in a discernible way through laboratory testing, it has progressed to the point where aggressive therapy is necessary. The solution to all this is a form of preventive medicine wherein each person takes the best possible care of him or herself through attention to whole, healthful foods entering his or her body.

Junk Food Addicts—The Effects on Our Children

All the same, why should this generation of human beings be the sacrificial lambs for the future generation of non-food eaters? If people take care of themselves now when this is just starting to happen, it follows that their future generations will have stronger constitutions and be able to deal more successfully with diseases and pollutants in the food supply.

Perhaps the most disturbing aspect of the lack of nutrition in this country has yet to be seen. There is a generation being raised right now on artificial colors, flavors, salt, refined sugar, bleached flour, chemicals, preservatives, and a whole array of synthetic additives. What will they—the infants and toddlers of today—be like when they reach adulthood and begin to reproduce? It could be that the most nutritious thing they have ever ingested was their mother's milk, even though *that* could have been full of additives from the mother's system as well.

Will we see a generation of Americans whose teeth rot out by the time they reach thirty, where a small outbreak of plague or disease could virtually wipe out entire cities, where people marry of necessity before the age of sixteen because they cannot be assured of the ability to reproduce much after that? Will their basic constitutions be capable of reproducing at all?

It may be tragic enough that most of the adult population is addicted to refined sugar, table salt, cola, and low-nutrition foods such as bleached flour, polished rice, and the whole array of additives and preservatives, but the most horrible and criminal aspect of this situation is the effect it will all have on our children.

Childrens' taste buds and food preferences are formed in infancy. Their addictions are established by the time they start elementary school. Improper nutrition results in weakened and deficient cellular structure, which is the very basis of life. Perhaps it's no wonder that so many of our school-age children have learning difficulties, or are hyperactive, bored, anxious, or have behavior problems. It could all stem from their diets!

Think twice the next time you are about to put a bottle of cola in your grocery cart, or yield to the kids' nagging for sweets or highly processed junk food. Take every opportunity to feed your children the most nutritious, healthful foods available. If you won't do it for yourself, the very least you can do is make sure that your children are healthy. When they are very young, they will never develop cravings or addictions to Coke, or Kool-Aid, or candy, or Wonder Bread unless you give it to them the first time.

It is really wonderful that parents of today are taking such an active interest in the natural birth process so that their infants may be born without drugs. Another good sign is that more and more mothers are choosing to breast-feed their infants to provide them with the natural immunities to disease and illness. But why should the caring and concern stop there? If you had your children through natural childbirth, there's no reason to resist the "natural way" for the rest of their lives.

If your children are already hooked on junk food (and it is interesting to point out here that a slang word for the killer drug heroin is "junk"), don't despair. You can still guide them away from the harmful things in their diets slowly and gradually. Children are very receptive to new ideas and new things, especially if you approach it correctly. It won't be a particularly easy process, but if your whole family can work at it together, it can be a very happy, rewarding experience for all of you. Once you begin to rid your systems of harmful substances, you may find that certain behavioral problems in children will disappear, particularly moodiness and hyperactivity.

Another important point to be made here is that the time to start thinking about having healthy children is before you even conceive them. Give yourself and your spouse at least twelve months of healthy, nutritious eating before beginning a new human being. Give your children every chance in the world to be the healthiest people they can be.

The tremendous increase in the incidence of cancer in this country is one of the most alarming aspects of national health. The American

Cancer Society states that cancer is so widespread that one in every four people will develop a malignancy during his or her lifetime. These figures are understandably frightening.

Some of the ways you can protect yourself from this dreaded disease is to take care of your body through nutrition, relaxation, and exercise. Most physicians will agree that the definition of a healthy body is one that is best able to fight off disease. Regardless of whether or not you can accept the idea that cancer may be linked to improper nutrition, you might accept the fact that a healthy body will have a better chance of warding off the unhealthy cell growth which is the beginning of cancer.

Insecticides

One of the most important ways to help yourself is to diminish the amount of toxins you ingest. Allowing your organs to perform their normal duties of producing beneficial enzymes, co-enzymes, and other nutrients that they can produce for themselves naturally when not over-loaded with substances to detoxify is the best method.

To give you an example of some of the toxins you may be unknowingly ingesting, consider the difference between a regular, scrubbed baked potato and potato chips. Potato chips go through several different processing steps and have approximately twenty additives inserted into them in production. A baked potato, with its skin, has not been processed. It is a potato, plain and simple.

The following are just two of the many products we consume that are subject to pesticide spraying. The list shows some of the legal insecticides that are used. Exactly which ones are used on any one particular piece of fruit is, of course, open to conjecture.

APPLES:
    Aldrin—0.25 ppm
    Bacillus Thuringiensis Berliner—exemption
    Benzene Hexachloride—5 ppm
    2—(p-tert-Butylphenoxy)—Isopropyl-2-ChloroethylSulfite-zero
    Captan—100 ppm
    Chlorbenside—3 ppm (including its sulfoxide and sulfone oxidation products)
    Chlordane—0.3 ppm
    p-Chlorophenyl Phenyl Sulfone—8 ppm
    1,1 bis (p-Chlorophenyl)-2,2,2-Trichloroethanol—5 ppm

S-(p-Cholorophenylthiomethyl) 0, 0,-Diethyl Phosphorodithioate—0.8 ppm
DDT—7 ppm
Demeton—0.75 ppm
Diasinon—0.75 ppm
Dichlone—3 ppm
2,4-Dichlorophenoxy Acetic Acid—5 ppm
Dicyclohexylamine Salt of Dinitro-o-Cyclohexylphenol—1 ppm
Dieldrin—0.25 ppm
0,0-Dimenthyl S-(4-oxo-1,2,3-Benzotriazin-3(4H)Ylmethyl) Phosphorodithioate—2 ppm
Dodine—5 ppm
EPN—3 ppm
Ethion—1 ppm
Ethozyquin—3 ppm
Ethyl 4, 4'-Dichlorobenzilate—5 ppm
Ethylene—exemption
Ferbam—7 ppm
Glyodin—5 ppm
Heptachlor and heltachlor Epoxide—zero Hexahydro 6, 9-Methano-2,4, 3-Benzodioxathiepin-3-oxide 6,7,8,9,10,10-Hexacholoro-1,5,5a,6,9,9a;2 ppm
Lead Arsenate—7 ppm
Lindane—10 ppm
Malathion—8 ppm
Maneb—7 ppm
Maganous Dimethyldithiocarbamate—7 ppm
Mercaptobenzothiazole—0.1 ppm
1-Methozycarbonyl-1-propen-2-yl Dimenthyl Phosphate and its Beta Isomer—0.5 ppm
Methozyclor—14 ppm
Methyl Bromide as inorganic Bromide—5 ppm
Napthalene Acetic Acid—1 ppm
Nicotine-containing compounds—2 ppm
Ovex— 3 ppm
Parathion—1 ppm
Phenothiazine—7 ppm
Sodium 2,2-Dichloropropionate—3 ppm
Sodium o-Phenylphenate—25 ppm
TDE—7 ppm
Thiram—7 ppm
Toxaphene—7 ppm
Zineb—7 ppm
Ziram—7 ppm

ON APPLES!!! You can see the need for organically grown foods.

Now let's look at cucumber:

CUCUMBER
  Aldrin—0.25 ppm
  Benzene Hexachloride—5 ppm
  2-(p-tert-Butylphenoxy)-Isopropyl-2-Chloroethyl Sulfite—zero
  Calcium Arsenate—3.5 ppm of combined As_2O_3
  Captan—100 ppm
  Chlorodane—0.3 ppm
  1,1-bis (p-Chlorophenyl) -2,2,2-Trichloroethanol—5 ppm
  S-(p-Chlorophenylthiomethyl) 0,0-Diethyl Phosphorodithioate—0.8 ppm
  DDT—7 ppm
  Diazinon—0.75 ppm
  Dieldrin—0.25 ppm
  Endrin—zero
  Ethylene Dibromide as inorganic Bromide—30 ppm
  Ferbam—7 ppm
  Lindane—10 ppm
  Malathion—8 ppm
  Maneb—7 ppm
  1-Methoxycarbonyl-1-Propen-2-yl Dimenthyl Phosphate and its Beta Isomer—0.25 ppm
  Methoxychlor—14 ppm
  Methyl Bromide as inorganic Bromide—30 ppm
  Nicotene-containing compounds—2 ppm
  Parathion—1 ppm
  TDE—7 ppm
  Toxaphene—7 ppm
  Zineb—7 ppm
  Ziram—7 ppm

This is one very good reason why organic fruits and vegetables are stressed throughout the Total Glow program. If you simply cannot find organic food suppliers in your area, consider growing your own. If this, too, is impossible, at least scrub your fresh fruits and vegetables with cider vinegar (organic, without preservatives), to help remove some of the toxins. Some people scrub them with Dr. Bronner's castile soap and then rinse well. Don't use chlorox as has been sometimes proposed. It is too toxic.

Athough some guidelines regarding the amounts of insecticides, and the times during which the plants may be sprayed, exist, the FDA staff is underpowered and only a small percentage of their staff, (perhaps one or two percent) is involved in enforcement of such efforts.[7]

[7]Ibid.

Are You A Food Faddist?

Who, really, are the food faddists? Is it the person who eats everything that your grandparents ate (including fertile eggs and home-grown vegetables) or are the faddists the people who ingest hundreds of things every year that are comprised almost entirely of preservatives, insecticides, additives, and other poisons?

One of the most interesting examples that comes to mind when discussing this area of food faddism is a vegetable known to all—the potato. Is the food faddist the person who prefers a baked potato with the skin intact, who eats the skin containing all the nutrients, vitamins, and minerals? Or is the food faddist the person who eats potato chips that have gone through twenty processing steps and have had approximately 18 additives put into them? If you compare the plain baked potato with what you might choose on your own to add flavor, which person do you think is the food faddist?

It is my contention that the people who are addicted to refined sugar, refined salt, bleached flour, additives, preservatives, and other poisons, and who let these things rule their lives and their emotions are the faddists. But don't dare go so far as to tell them that, unless you want to make enemies.

Sometimes we know when we are hurting ourselves, and at other times we don't. Ask any smoker if he/she would like to quit, and the resoundingly high percentage will say, "YES! Of course I want to quit smoking!" Ask any person who has just finished bingeing on sweets or processed snacks how he feels, and he will probably tell you he feels terrible.

It won't do you any good to lecture them or try to make them feel guilty or any worse than they already do. Most people come to a realization one day that they are going to do a complete turn-around and start taking better care of themselves. Perhaps this is the point you had reached when you picked up this book. But most of us haven't the slightest idea where to begin.

So if you really want to help yourself, your friends, and your family, don't lecture or come on too strongly about healthy foods. Slowly broach the subject. It is so controversial that many have already made up their minds that healthy foods aren't any better than junk food. Gradually offer them some of the delicious new foods you are eating. If you push too hard or come on too strong, you're riding for a fall, and they will resent you. Just remember how you might have felt the first time you heard about natural foods. Didn't the subject bring hippies, communes, oriental mysteries, and other unfamiliar and threatening images to mind?

Try to respect the fact that everyone has a right to believe what he/she wants to believe, and has a right to make his/her own decisions. As much as you care about another person, you may not violate those rights just as you would not want your rights to be impinged upon. Hopefully, someday we will all be eating, exercising, and relaxing ourselves. Wouldn't that be a beautiful world in which to live? One way you might broach the subject is to tell them about the Total Glow program and buy them a copy of this book. If the book is a gift, they might be more responsive.

Helping Your Body Do Its Job

The importance of caring for the organs of the body that are mainly responsible for detoxification is something that few of us ever think about. These organs are primarily the liver, kidneys, skin, colon, and lungs. Most of us tend to take these organs for granted.

Consider the whole process of digestion of food. The digestive process begins in the mouth where chewing and saliva combine to break the food into manageable size. The stomach and intestinal tract then digest and absorb the nutrients into the blood stream, where it reaches individual blood cells. There the nutrients are metabolized into energy, water, carbon dioxide, and waste materials.

If the body is unable to convert much of the food into energy, water, and carbon dioxide, a great percentage of it becomes waste, which has to be eliminated for a healthy state to be maintained. As waste materials accumulate, they begin to interfere with the normal functioning of the cells. The cells will continue to produce metabolic debris and the blood then carries it to the organs that detoxify it.

Obviously, if these organs are already over-loaded and filled with debris, as is often the case with the colon, then the detoxification of further "leftovers" will be hugely slowed or completely impossible. In this case, the individual cells begin to accumulate debris. It gets reabsorbed from such areas as the small and large intestine to the extent that these organs become filled with mucus. This then makes it doubly difficult for nutrients to pass through in the normal way and be used by your body. It tends to have a snow-ball effect, until the beneficial nutrients are blocked and eliminated, and the poisons just keep circulating around in the bloodstream.

To give a graphic illustration of the process, think back to the garbage strike in New York City. Imagine that the City is the human body, and that all the residents are individual cells. The garbage collectors are the body's detoxification organs, and the garbage dumps and barges are the waste elimination systems.

If the garbage collectors strike and refuse to collect the garbage, it sits around on the streets and festers. The individual cells keep putting their garbage out to be collected, but it sits there and the piles get bigger every day. Disease spreads from the rotting garbage. The individual cells become weak, but they still keep eliminating their garbage, trying to get rid of it. When the garbage collectors finally *do* go back to work, the dumps and river barges are completely clogged, making the elimination of the waste virtually impossible. It may be months or years until the system is finally operating at peak efficiency again.

In the case of New York, there was a quickly noticeable effect, but such is not the case with our bodies. Frequently, it can take years of abuse before the degeneration makes itself apparent.

Though somewhat shocking, the above illustration is given to provide you with an idea of what harmful foods can do when they collect in your body and are not eliminated. It's definitely something worth thinking about, isn't it? Although it is truly amazing sometimes what the body can tolerate, it can never do you any harm to start paying attention to the kinds of foods you are putting into it. Raw fruits and vegetables are the main things that will help you assist your detoxification organs, along with whole grains, bran, unpolished rice, and other natural, unprocessed foods.

Your Skin—And How to Care for It.

The skin is a vitally important detoxification organ. Usually, it is the last organ to be called upon when the other organs are bogged down, and when signs of abuse start showing in your skin, it's a good indication that things have gone too far and that it is time to change. The tell-tale signs are eruptions, blemishes, changes in color, severe to moderate acne, psoriasis, wrinkles at a premature age, and a host of other problems. Though things like eczema and other rashes are directly or indirectly related to stress, most other skin problems are caused by toxins that have accumulated in the body.

Your skin is a very good barometer for you to use in judging your overall health, especially if you are an adult. While hormonal changes frequently cause acne in adolescents, adult acne is an entirely different story. The extent to which these things continue and persist is a signal indicating the fact that something else is probably not functioning well in your body.

Sometimes it is interesting to think back to some advice our mothers gave us about the ways in which our bodies functioned. It is especially interesting that people seem to know somehow inside of themselves what is right and what is harmful when it comes to food. Do you remember your mother telling you that the little sore spots you got in your mouth meant that your stomach was upset?

Many cultures even have their own rituals that they observe in regard to eating meals. Consider the Jewish rules about separating the meat and dairy dishes and utensils. Even animals seem to know when something is out of kilter. Cats and dogs, especially, will go off their food and eat grass (or house plants!) until they vomit or somehow rid themselves of what they know is making them ill. They are instinctively intelligent enough to let their bodies rest and stop eating for awhile. We could learn alot from our pets.

If people can teach themselves to again be able to recognize their bodies' warning signals, it will be a great step in the right direction. Others have reported certain cravings for food like fish or fruit or carrots. This, in its simplest and most primitive form, is your body telling you what it needs. Pay attention to the signals.

Another indication of our ignorance of our bodies comes from the ways in which we care for our skin. When we develop outbreaks or dry skin, we immediately run to the drugstore to buy the latest chemical preparation to clear it up. Women spend millions of dollars annually on night creams, wrinkle creams, soaps, astringents, hair conditioners, facials, masks, moisturizers, and a variety of other preparations that guarantee a more beautiful complexion. Isn't it amazing that no one stops to think that beauty starts from within (an inner glow), and that no matter what you slap or plaster onto the outside of your skin, it isn't going to make much difference if you are basically unhealthy underneath it all?

If you want to have clear skin that seems to glow from underneath, that appears to be radiantly healthy and free from dryness, oiliness, blemishes, and other problems, start paying attention to what you are feeding it through your mouth.

The skin has been called the "third kidney" and is a breathing organ. Perhaps if you think in those terms, you will be more inclined to take good care of it. To begin with, the best way to care for your skin is to eat the right foods. Because the skin is one of the last organs in the body to receive nutrients, it responds the latest. If you have a problem like psoriasis, a difficult acne situation, neuro-dematitis, or any of a whole class of different problems, it is very important for you to understand that healthy eating will play a determining role in conquering these ailments.

Saunas

Another possibility to consider is saunas and practices that will stimulate your skin. Again, check with your doctor if you have any suspicions about heart trouble before undertaking any of the following suggestions.

Saunas help stimulate the skin and aid in the elimination of mucous in the body. After taking a sauna bath, step into a cool shower. Your skin will feel tingly and alive immediately. Purchase a loofah sponge and/or natural brush that you can use to rub away dead skin cells. In the shower, go from hot to cool several times.

Some other suggestions would be to avoid using aluminum-based and hexachlorophene-type products. Plain water and a good brush, with some natural soap, are all you really need. Another nice thing you can do for the skin is to take a luxurious bath for five or ten minutes in warm water to which you have added about a cup of natural apple cider vinegar. This will maintain your natural acid/alkaline balance which your skin needs to stay healthy. Once you have finished bathing, dry yourself vigorously with a towel until you feel tingly and warm all over. Don't overdo it, though, as you are just trying to stimulate and rub off some of the dead cells, not damage tender skin in any way.

Getting your skin working again will be refreshing and provide you with an inner glow of beauty that all the cosmetics in the world will not be able to duplicate.

Dry Brush Massage

As mentioned previously, the skin has been grossly overlooked in its importance in eliminating body waste material. Under chemical analysis, the composition of perspiration shows a high content of uric acid (a metabolic waste product), which is also a component in urine.

When the pores of the skin become choked and filled with debris and dead cells, the powerful waste eliminating ability of the skin is impaired. The consequence is that more work is required by the kidneys and liver.

In a body with a heavy skin layer, approximately a pound of waste matter can be expelled through it daily. From the Finnish saunas (of my own ancestry) to the ancient Roman baths, one can see the early understanding of the healing powers of sweating, and as a method of caring for the skin and the entire body.

Skin also absorbs various vitamins and minerals. Through sunlight on our bodies, we absorb Vitamin D, which is important to our health.

Therefore, I highly recommend a dry brush massage to rejuvenate and help your entire body on the road to maintaining and improving your overall health.

Increased blood circulation occurs during massage, especially in the small blood vessels of the skin and in the underlying organs and muscles. Removal of the dead cells and other impurities helps keep the pores open and stimulates the glands located in the skin. Your complexion will naturally improve and you will feel healthier sooner.

Purchase a natural fiber brush with a long handle so that you can reach all parts of your body. Try to get a good brush about two or three inches in diameter or roughly the size of your hand. Be sure it is made of natural fibers, as many of the synthetic fibers will be too harsh for your skin. As many of these brushes are foreign made, I suggest a loofah sponge in the meantime to get started.

Loofahs, which are coarse natural sponges, come in the forms of mittens, long plain pieces, or longer strips with plastic handles on either end. The latter facilitates reaching your back. I recommend using the loofah while bathing and the dry brush afterwards. For hygenic reasons, each member of your family should have their own brush. Wash and dry them every two or three weeks, as debris collects inside them.

Facial skin is very sensitive, so I would not recommend using the sponge or brush there. Also, don't brush on an area where there is an infection. Start with the soles of your feet and brush circularly all the way up the backs of your legs to your buttocks, up your back, and then up the front of your body and legs. Start brushing gently and apply pressure, according to your sensitivity. Next start at your palms and go up that side of your arm and down the other. These motions facilitate the natural blood flow.

There really isn't any strict pattern to your brushing, and you may even find it enjoyable to do it with your partner and brush each other. It's a pleasant way of giving and taking, and can put you in greater touch with your own body as well as your partner's.

Oil Massage

Another nice thing you can do for your skin is to massage it with a nutritious oil. A suggestion would be:
>   3 or 4 tablespoons olive oil
>   6 or 8 tablespoons sesame oil
>   2 tablespoons almond oil
>   a few drops of perfume, if desired

Pour these ingredients into an empty glass bottle and shake well. Store in the refrigerator and use a few drops daily. If you have dry skin, apply to your face, neck, and hands. Treat your whole body to an oil rub at least once a week.

Making your own cosmetics in this manner is quick and easy, and lots of fun. Natural, home-made cosmetics are the healthiest in preventing wrinkles and the aging of your skin. I would tend to believe that they are less expensive, too.

Your Liver And Your Life

The word "liver" means life, and there probably isn't another word that could describe it better. The thousands of tasks performed daily by our livers is astounding. It is involved in the metabolism of all major food groups, the breakdown of most medical drugs, the storage of foods, the detoxification process, and is involved in crucial enzyme reactions our bodies need to perform to keep us alive. A healthy liver is essential to a healthy you.

There are some very basic things you can do to help your liver do its job. Pay attention to what you eat. A balanced, nutritious diet is essential. Don't overload your liver with extra toxins to break down. White flour, for example, is hard on your liver, so substitute whole grain breads that supply it with the natural support it needs. Keep the amount of additives and preservatives you eat to absolute minimum, since most of these have to be detoxified by the liver.

Take only prescription drugs directed by your physician. It may be a good idea to purchase a prescription encyclopedia so that you will know which drugs should not be taken together, their effects, etc. An occasional aspirin or aspirin substitute is not going to hurt you, but pay closer attention to remedies and over-the-counter preparations, which have to be handled by your liver.

Keep alcoholic consumption to a minimum. I don't want to go overboard in this area, because many people enjoy a glass of wine or a cocktail on occasion. But start to watch yourself more closely if you notice a tendency to over-indulge. Moderation is the answer. Of course, for many, eliminating alcohol completely is the only answer, and I would question even the most moderate use of alcohol by anyone who has cancer. In addition to alcohol being bad for your liver, it is not made as well as it was years ago. Beer is a good example. It used to be made with great care and constant supervision. Then came the addition of refined sugar to augment the fermentation process and with it came a decrease in the quality of the beverage.

As mentioned in the section on supplementing your diet, the use of Brewer's Yeast, which is rich in vitamins, is advisable, along with a new type of more potent yeast called "mega-yeast."

For those of you who are interested in more intensive liver information, such as fasting, enemas, liver purges, and liver flushes, I suggest:

"How to Stay Slim, Healthy, and Young with Juice Fasting" by Dr. Paavo Airola, and *"One Answer to Cancer,"* by Dr. William Kelley.

Both are available at most health food stores or they will order them for you. Be sure to check with your doctor before fasting.

The liver is one organ that rejuvenates itself with proper care, where this is not the case with most other organs. Take good care of your liver—it's one of the most important organs in your body.

Don't Blame The Doctors If They Don't Know

Speaking personally as a physician, I have always been bothered by the schism I experienced in my own medical training. This concerned the separation of the body and mind, where doctors who concentrate on the physical aspects of medicine seem to be totally separated from those being trained in psychiatry.[8]

Throughout the history of medicine, this separation has existed and bitter battles have been fought. Obviously, some of this conflict was positive, as it made doctors re-examine their thinking, made them work harder to learn more so that they could increasingly help their patients. Patients and colleagues are constantly challenging physicians to examine what they know, think, and how it eventually effects them.

In the same way that psychiatry has been cut off from the mainstream of medicine, so has nutrition. The idea of teaching about food, the ways in which it is used and how it effects the body, and the

---

[8]Roger J. Williams, *Nutrition Against Disease* (New York: Pittman Publishing Co., 1971).

ways in which to prepare nutritious meals, has been left to Home Economics departments. Here, the subject is considered less of a science and more of an area of useful knowledge for home makers to use along with sewing, cleaning, and child care. It is hard to find any scientists majoring in Home Economics, and (interestingly enough) this is one course of study which has been phased out of most college curriculums.

Dieticians, of course, are medical professionals who have been trained in the effects of different diets for different diseases. Yet it would be difficult, if not impossible, to find a dietician versed in the diets that could *prevent* the onset of these diseases. Their training emphasis is on diets used after the diseases have occurred.

Very few medical schools offer courses on the subject of nutrition in their medical curriculums. Of the less than one-third of the schools that do offer these courses, the accentuation and the time given to the subject is very minimal.[9]

The doctors being trained today in the large number of medical schools in this country have some of the best training that has ever been offered. But they are practicing now on bodies of patients that are not in as good a condition as they were several years ago when the textbooks were written. Most doctors in our country are now practicing crisis medicine. We really can't be expected to repair your slipped disc, ulcer, or cystic breast disease overnight when the underlying causes may be based in poor nutrition; which is an area where we have not been trained. Doctors are being presented with bodies that have taken years to get into the poor health they are in now, and sometimes they no longer respond to antibiotics and medications that are administered. I believe that we must build up our own bodies so that we can respond better to the treatments that physicians have to offer.

As mentioned before, modern physicians are practicing crisis medicine. With all of their expertise and brilliance today, the majority do not know enough about nutrition. Before problems show up on many of the classical medical tests, the condition will have already reached the point where aggressive treatment is necessary. In a liver test, for example, before the results show abnormality, the liver may be operating at only twenty to fifty percent of its ability. For certain other organs, namely the pancreas and adrenals, we have no early-warning tests.

The human body is so miraculous that it can readily make up for

---

[9]Carlton Fredericks, *Look Younger, Feel Healthier,* Op. Cit. and *The Wall Street Journal,* "Worldwide News" June 13, 1978.

deficiencies, for a time. For instance, if we are low in potassium and calcium, it will take calcium from our bones and gastro-intestinal tracts to replace what is missing in the blood. Minerals like calcium can greatly effect our emotional states. It can cause us to awaken with leg cramps and have difficulty with menstrual cycles, etc. But even if a general calcium test seems to be all right, it does not mean that you don't need more of that particular element. The calcium showing up in your blood test might have been extracted from your teeth and bones.

So it would be wise to take the best care possible of those organs that do not show damage readily on standard tests and examinations. Although this discussion is in no way an attempt to discredit modern medicine and its practitioners, it *is* a call to professionals and non-professionals alike to begin paying greater attention to the more simpler truths in life. Let us start looking at the real causes of disease and malfunction where they originate.

It may be a good idea for you to discuss some of these ideas with your personal physician. It could be an eye-opening experience for him or her. Remember that they didn't learn much about nutrition in medical school because there simply wasn't enough time. Go easy on your doctors if they don't seem to be interested at first. They really do care about you, and once they start seeing the improvement you are making in your health through efforts in nutrition, relaxation, and exercise, they will be overjoyed.

This area, along with relaxation and exercise, is a whole new realm of investigation that has long been ignored or left to the non-professionals. Once medicine becomes involved in these areas, progress toward eliminating the many crippling or fatal diseases will be greatly facilitated.

Nutrition And Having A Baby

The importance of proper nutrition before pregnancy is never greater. I believe that it involves both partners in the relationship, not the mother to the exclusion of the father. The father's diet prior to conception has been virtually ignored. Even so, most mothers don't give it a second thought until they are already pregnant. That is the time when they start taking vitamin supplements, quit smoking, eliminate alcohol, and stay away from drugs. This is fine, but the time to start doing these things, along with eating the healthiest food available, is about twelve months before the baby is even conceived.

This applies to the father as well, since he provides one complete half of the conceived fetus. Following the basic nutritional outlines in this book will be of immense benefit to both the mother and father, not to mention the future child. That, of course, includes organically grown foods to the extent that you can obtain them, eating green vegetables daily, incorporating the salads and dressings offered in this book, whole grain cereals and breads, milk, and eating two fertile eggs (lightly poached) each day. The protein in the eggs can help conteract any pregnancy-related feelings of dizziness, confusion, inability to concentrate, nervousness, or lethargy you might be experiencing.

Try to eat more of the organ foods such as sweet breads, liver, tripe, shad roe, kidneys, and heart. Although these things are quite strongly flavored, if you add a bit to your ground meats, you will eventually develop a taste for them. (I make my meatloaf with half heart and half hamburger. No one detects the heart, and they love the recipe.) These meats are marvelous sources of iron, protein, and minerals. It might help you to remember that some of the healthiest natives on earth commonly eat these organs first when they have killed an animal, and literally throw the flesh and muscle meat (including filet mignon) to the dogs. Again, this is an example of the inherent wisdom of folk traditions.

Avoid pastries, ice cream, candies, and desserts, especially anything made with refined sugar. Reference is made again to *Sugar Blues*, a book so powerful, well-documented and convincing that it may very well change your entire life.

Take the supplements that your doctor prescribes, but add extra liver capsules, a multiple vitamin and mineral capsule, brewer's yeast, and Vitamin E. These supplements supply the Vitamin B-complex, iodine, and many of the necessary minerals not found in American diets. All these things can be found in your health food store in natural form. While synthetic vitamins may be better than nothing at all, natural vitamins are best.

The Role of the Father

To illustrate the importance of the father's diet prior to conception, the following study is presented:

> Weston Price recounts an experiment in dogs in which he mated a well-nourished male dog with four well-nourished female dogs, producing four litters of normal puppies.
>
> The same male was then fed an inadequate diet and re-mated with the same four well-fed females to produce four litters that were deformed to a large extent.

> *The deformed males of these litters were then given good diets and re-mated with the same group of well-nourished females from the litters. The result was four normal litters.*
>
> *Despite the fact that medical people have used frogs to diagnose pregnancy, and cats to measure the importance of digitalis, there was a criticism of the validity of this test with the dogs, saying that one cannot leap from conclusions about dogs and apply them as conclusions about humans!*[10]

The problem has been that we have been paying far too little attention to men and their role in child bearing. If I were of the male sex, I would feel somewhat cheated. Hopefully someday, men will be given as much recognition in the reproduction of normal, healthy babies as women are given now. If a pregnancy is not normal, on the other hand, usually it is the mother's "fault." If she fails to conceive, miscarries, or delivers an abnormal child, consciously or unconsciously, she accepts the blame.

As a psychiatrist, I have also seen men who are victims of subconsciously blaming themselves for an unsuccessful pregnancy in their wives. I do hope the day will come when couples prepare together for healthy babies by making themselves as healthy as possible beforehand.

Equal obscurity has been given to the research of Wilfred Chute, in which he demonstrated that nutritional treatment of fathers prior to conception resulted in a drop in the incidence of deformity of babies born to mothers having a previous record of giving birth to deformed babies. Statistically speaking, mothers with a history of bearing deformed babies face a greater probability of such diasters than do mothers whose previous babies were normal.

Chute gave Vitamin E to the fathers of such children prior to the next conception. There was a drop of approximately 84% in the anticipated number of abnormalities in subsequent pregnancies. A type of research control was offered in the following way: not only was there a record of the mother's previous abnormal births, but subsequently (in certain instances) the father discarded the Vitamin E regimen. In those cases, the incidence of deformity in pregnancy rose to its former level.[11]

The Well-fed Baby

If you already have a baby or are expecting one soon, you can do one of the greatest things ever. Begin feeding it well or start now to

---
[10] Carlton Fredericks, *Look Young, Feel Healthier*, Op. Cit.
[11] Ibid.

feed it well. Following the basic guidelines in this book, you can have a happy, healthy baby.

Start by making your own baby food. If you must buy commercially prepared baby food, read the labels and know what you are feeding your child. *Avoid the sugar and salt addictions* that are started in infancy through commercial products. Let your infant enjoy his or her taste buds before they become numbed to all tastes by sugar and salt. Don't subject your baby to your addictions and the years spent kicking the habit. Remember that any addiction results in a decreased resistance to disease. Allow your child to grow up healthy.

Cancer: The Possible Causes

If there was one disease on earth that you had the power to cure, which one would it be? Most frequently, the answer to that question is "cancer." Increasingly, people fear what has been called by many "the Big C." Although heart disease and cancer are the two main killers in America, people fear cancer the most. They feel helpless, don't know what they can do to prevent it, and fear that it can strike at almost any time. Some even put off having physical exams, thinking that the longer they can go without knowing about it, the easier it will be.

Once cancer was relegated to older people in their 60's and 70's, with the exception of such malignancies as Hodgkins Disease and certain leukemias, which strike the young. Now cancer is appearing almost everywhere, at anytime, and it is not selective about who it hits. Rarely a week passes when we do not learn of a friend or acquaintance (some even as young as their early 20's) who are victims of this frightening disease.

I believe that it's time we re-evaluate our thinking in terms of understanding cancer, its causes, and cures. Even prominent medical journals are calling for this, as was indicated in the April, 1978 issue of the Journal of Surgery, Gynecology, and Obstetrics.

My personal feelings are that probably no *one* thing causes cancer in all cases, especially not in the epidemic proportions we are witnessing today. The cumulative effect of a great many things is probably the major reason for the increase in cancer. This would include things we are eating, breathing, and being exposed to in various forms. Our bodies could probably handle some of these stresses, but not all of them, and not all at once. We cannot physically adapt to so many changes so quickly.

Listed below are some of the possible causes of cancer as discussed

Day 3 Eating For Your Health And Happiness 141

by the leading medical and nutritional researchers in the country. Obviously, as time progresses, we will discover more causes. In the "Suggested Readings" section of this book, I have listed several sources where you will find more thought and further research on the subject. Here are the current theories. Try to keep them in mind.

1. **Excessive smoking.**
2. **Water.** Certain chemicals are added to our water supply to counteract the increased amount of pollutants.[12]
3. **Diethylstilbesterol.** This is a hormone injected into beef cattle and other livestock to fatten and hasten their growth.
4. **Nitrorosamines.** Nitrates and nitrites found in many sandwich meats, ham, and hot dogs. Also found in smoked fish (the Japanese, who consume large quantities of smoked fish have a high incidence of stomach cancer).[13]
5. **Irritation.** Mechanical and physical, as in pipe smoking.
6. **Stontium 90.** Radioactive fallout from atomic testing and explosions.
7. **Overeating, Excess Drinking, Too Many Fats.** In *The Challenge of Cancer*, published by the National Cancer Institute, it stated, "There is statistical evidence from various insurance companies that overweight persons have a distinctly greater tendency for developing cancer." Dr. Arthur Upton, Director of the National Cancer Institute, told a Senate subcommittee that the institute would do more to tell people that there is already strong evidence that three types of dietary abuse—overeating, excess drinking, and too many fats in the diet may lead to cancer.[14]
8. **Lack of Fiber in Diet.** The colons (large intestine) of most people in this country are clogged and sluggish. Our overcooked or processed food, lack of fresh produce and raw vegetables, lack of fiber and grains in our diet has helped to produce this condition. It is noteworthy that the incidence of cancer of the colon has dramatically increased in the last twenty years. A link between this and improper nutrition exists, in my opinion. A study affirming this was released from the University of Illinois at Urbana, stating that a link be-

---
[12]*The Wall Street Journal,* June 13, 1978.
[13]*Newsweek,* "Cancer and Our Diet." June 24, 1978.
[14]Victor Conn, "How Diet Effects Cancer Newest Target on Institute," *The Washington Post,* June 14, 1978.

tween cancer of large intestine and the lack of fiber in our diets does exist.[15]
9. **Smog.**
10. **High Estrogen Levels.** This, coupled with the lowered ability of the liver to metabolize estrogen to estriol, leads to breast cancer. Tremendously powerful, well-documented case presented by Carlton Fredericks in his book, *Breast Cancer–A Nutritional Approach.*
11. **Hexachlorophene.** Found in many cosmetics, deodorants, and soaps.[16]
12. **Rancid Food and Oils.**[17]
13. **Improper Diet and Poor Nutrition.**[18]
14. **Excessive X-rays.**
15. **Inability to Metabolize Proteins.** Inability to utilize, break down, and excrete the by-products of protein.[19]
16. **Stress.**[20]
17. **Salt.**[21]
18. **Cadmium.** Present in phosphate fertilizers in excess, taken up by and concentrated in the liver of animals and shellfish.

You can begin to reduce your risk of getting cancer by bearing the preceding list in mind. Pay closer attention to the causes. Your diet alone probably contains many of the listed items, so try to avoid these things. By keeping a daily log of what you eat, you will be surprised at the toxins you are accumulating.

Let's take, for example, a submarine or hoagie sandwich, which is a popular lunch item in many parts of the country. The hoagie probably has several lunch meats with nitrites and nitrates, there may be food coloring in the cheese, preservatives in the roll and dressings, and the vegetables were probably sprayed with insecticides (none of which we

---

[15] *The Washington Post,* June 3, 1978, and *Newsweek,* "Cancer and Our Diet," Op. Cit.
[16] Paavo Airola, Ph.D., N.D., *Cancer, The Total Approach* (Phoenix: Health Plus Publishers, 1972).
[17] *Let's Live,* November, 1977, and Richard Passwater, *Supernutrition* (New York: The Dial Press, 1975).
[18] *The Washington Post,* June 13, 1978.
[19] *Healthview Newsletter,* Vol. 1, No. 5, 1977, and William Donald Kelly, B.A., D.D.A., M.S., F.I.C.A.N., *One Answer to Cancer* (Beverly Hills: The Kelly Foundation, The International Association of Cancer Victims and Friends, Inc., 1969).
[20] Lawrence Le Shan, *Cancer and Personality: A Critical Review,* Op. Cit.
[21] Paavo Airola, Ph.D., N.D., *Cancer, The Total Approach,* Op. Cit.

know to be safe). Add a cola or some soft drink, and you've got refined sugar, artificial colorings, and artificial flavorings, plus the chemicals to make it carbonated. If you have French fries or potato chips, you have added the possibility of rancid oil to your lunch, not to mention the additives and preservatives present. Most oils are heated to high temperatures and go through an oxidation process whereby harmful substances are produced within the oil, termed "cancer-causing free radicals."[22] The important aspect is that a heavy consumption of these polyunsaturated oils (which are low in Vitamin E, a natural antioxidant), can lead to cancer. A balance between polyunsaturated and saturated fats is more appropriate.

A large number of studies alarmingly show proportionate increases in cancer (especially breast cancer) with increasing dietary polyunsaturate levels. This finding comes from epidemiological studies in several countries where considerable quantities of fish, and lesser quantities of eggs and dairy products, are consumed.[23]

Some foods that are most vunerable to rancidity are some of those previously thought of as health foods. These include whole wheat flour, wheat germ, sesame seeds, and oils. Wheat germ turns rancid within about a week. When foods become rancid, Vitamins E, A, and F are destroyed, and chemicals are released that can be cancer-causing. Dr. H. Aremueller of Germany, the foremost authority on rancidity in foods, acknowledges that this is so, and his findings are confirmed by Drs. Rownee and Burrett of the University of Pennsylvania.

When you buy whole wheat flour, obtain it from a store that grinds it daily, or "while you wait." Make your own bread with several friends, taking turns each month. You might also be able to find co-ops where people work together and grind wheat berries daily. Buying from these sources is safe, if you bake the bread within a few days of buying the flour. Because I am so fond of whole wheat bread, I decided to buy my own electric mill. They are not inexpensive (about $200), but perhaps you could share the cost with several friends.

How to Protect Yourself From Cancer

So there *are* answers to the problem of cancer. Never overeat. Decrease your salt intake. Use alcohol only in moderation. Decrease your refined sugar intake. Increase fiber, whole grains, and bran in your diet. Increase the ratio of raw foods in your diet. Work with the

---

[22]A. C. Ivy, *Gastroenterology,* March, 1955.
[23]Richard A. Passwater, *Supernutrition* (New York: The Dial Press, 1975).

Environmental Protection Agency to cut down on pollution of the air and water. Check your water supply for chemicals, and if dangerous levels are present, drink distilled water, tested spring water, or purified water. Teach yourself how to relax through meditation. Eliminate foods preserved with nitrites and nitrates. Balance the amount of polyunsaturates and saturated fats in your diet, exercise, and make and keep regular medical appointments and check ups.

The answers are endless. All it takes is that you become aware of what you are doing and take steps to improve the quality of your life.

Food Supplements: Why We Need Them

It is my opinion that supplementing the daily diet is crucial for the following reasons:

1. The detoxification organs (particularly the liver) need help, especially if we continue to ingest enormous amounts of toxins.

2. Modern food processing techniques remove virtually all (or most all) of the valuable and essential nutrients.

3. The soils in which commercial food is grown is gradually being depleted of its nutrient-giving qualities.

4. The elemental proto-plasm of people who have grown up on processed foods with additives, preservatives, and other toxins is weakened.

Supplements are not inexpensive, and many argue that most people do not assimilate the majority of them. If you turn the argument around, however, you will find that the small amount of money spent in taking care of yourself cannot come close to the current figures (of between $10,000 and $50,000 or more annually per person) for the treatment of cancer. It makes sense to begin caring for yourself in the most effective way possible, in order to help offset future potential disease and disability.

Although the subject of food supplements is a complicated one, and there are many different schools of thought, the following is presented as a basic outline. You are urged to do some of your own further research if the subject appeals to you, as it is a fascinating topic. See the Suggested Readings section for further information.

There are, of course, individual differences, and some people may benefit from more or less of a particular supplement. Also, it is generally more beneficial to take an entire program of supplements, as they work synergistically. You can take one of the B-complex vitamins alone, for example, but it may not work as well as it would if the whole complex of B Vitamins were ingested. Some vitamins taken alone could be harmful. Be careful. If you have questions, go over your program with your doctor or nutritionist.

I do want to emphasize, however, that supplements are just that—food supplements. They are not substitutes for good food, but rather an addition. They are necessary because it is difficult to obtain consistently healthful foods.

Which Ones We Need

A basic supplemental program for an adult or teenager would be the following:

Vitamin A—5,000 to 10,000 units daily, with meals
Vitamin D—400 to 800 units daily, with meals
Vitamin E—400 units daily, with meals
Vitamin C—250 to 2,000 units daily, with meals
Vitamin B-complex—one to three times daily, with meals
Flaxseed—minimum requirement not established*
Manganese—10 to 20 mgs. daily
Phosphorus—100 to 500 mgs. daily
Calcium—250 to 500 mgs. daily ⎫ may be taken in
Magnesium—100 to 200 mgs. daily ⎭ form of Dolomite
Zinc—50 to 100 mgs. daily
Iron—10 to 15 mgs. daily
Selenium—50 to 100 mcg. daily
Chromium—found in brewer's yeast 500 mcg. daily
Liver—2 to 4 vacuum-dried tablets twice daily, with meals
Adrenal supplement—1 to 2 raw concentrate tablets daily with meals
Pancreatic Enzyme (Enteric Coated) 1 to 4 tablets with meals **
Trace Minerals—1 tablet daily, with meals
Multiple Vitamins with Minerals—1 tablet daily, with meals
Dolomite (Calcium/magnesium)—100 to 200 mgs. daily
Iodine—0.10 to 0.20 mgs. daily
Lecithin—2½ grams daily (½ tablespoon). Take ½ tablespoon daily with a small glass of juice. When eating in a restaurant, take 2 capsules after each meal to help in the metabolism of fats.
Garlic—Kyolic Brand, 2 tablets, twice a day***

*Helps assimilation of Calcium
** Greatly aids in digestion of protein.

Kelp, Sea Salt, Bone Meal—excellent sources of trace minerals.

HCl Pepsin—1 tablet daily with meals****

Supplementing the liver, regardless of what vitamin supplements you take, is essential. Since the liver is the main organ of detoxifying our bodies, it needs all the support you can give it. Eating liver itself is valuable, but for non-liver eaters, here is a suggestion; there are vacuum-dried liver tablets available that are made from animals who have not been raised on DDT-sprayed foods or insecticides. Also read labels and be certain they are not dried at temperatures exceeding 37° C. Temperatures above this will destroy most of the important enzymes. This same rule applies to all organ supplements.

The following is a chart of the various vitamins, what they do for you, their natural sources, and the ways in which a deficiency makes itself known. By way of definition, the following explanations of the terms used in the chart are presented.

"Natural Sources"—the foods where these particular vitamins and minerals are found in their natural state.

"Biochemical Uses"—the ways in which your body uses these vitamins, why they are needed, and what they do.

"Flagrant Clinical Symptoms"—symptoms that are detectable by physicians, usually through clinical tests and observation.

"Non-detectable Clinical Symptoms"—symptoms for which there are no clinical or laboratory tests. These are conditions that perhaps only you will be able to detect and report to your physician.

"RDA Requirements"—the dosage amount determined by the Federal Government as a minimum daily requirement for maintaining health.

"Supplement Amount"—dosages that might be taken over and above the RDA Requirement.

"Possible Help in Disease and Prevention"—ways in which these vitamins and minerals can aid your body in its many functions.

"Toxicity"—amounts that should not be exceeded, symptoms of ingestion of large doses of particular vitamins or minerals. Toxicity and therapeutic amounts will naturally vary from individual to individual.

"Synergistic Effects"—the ways in which this vitamin reacts to other foods and vitamins.

"Danger of Using Alone"—possible or known complications of using a particular vitamin or mineral by itself.

*** If you have a tendency toward high blood pressure, take 2 tablets, 3 times a day.—From *The Miracle of Garlic,* Paavo Airola, Ph.D., N.D., Health Plus Publishers, Phoenix, AZ: 1978.

****If you have an ulcer, omit this.

Dr. Rona's Suggestions

Vitamin A — Retinol*

Natural Sources: Fish liver oil, carrots, green and yellow vegetables, liver, whole milk, dairy products, egg yolks, yellow fruits.

Biochemical Uses: Essential for growth and maintenance of body tissues, bones, teeth, and eyesight. Helps form and maintain healthy skin, hair, teeth, gums, glands, and mucous membranes.

Flagrant Clinical Symptoms: Night blindness (nyctalopia), thickening of the cornea of the eye (xerophthalmia), could cause ulceration and/or blindness.

Non-detectable Clinical Symptoms: Inability of eyes to adjust to darkness, dry and inflamed eyes, sties. Skin blemishes, roughness, premature aging, loss of smell, appetite. Fatigue, diarrhea dry/dull hair, dandruff, hair loss, poor nail condition.

RDA Requirements: 5,000 I.U. for adults and children over four years of age (Pregnant and lactating women 8,000 I.U.)

Supplement Amounts: 10,000 to 25,000 I.U. daily, therapeutic dose.

Possible Help in Disease and Prevention: Preventing pre-cancerous cells from becoming cancerous. Prevention of colds and other viruses. Effects development of teeth. Increases resistance to infection. Conditions the mucous membranes of the body. Nourishes skin and hair. Prevents eye diseases and night blindness. Helps digest proteins.

Toxicity: More than 50,000 I.U. could produce toxic effects (blurred vision, nausea, vomiting, dizziness, changes in bone, ligaments, tendons, and skin) and should only be taken under supervision of a medical doctor. Chronic ingestion of large amounts have been reported to cause disorders of liver function, psychiatric side-effects mimicking schizophrenia.

Synergistic Effect of this vitamin: Use with B2. Helps to prevent/correct cataracts and improves health of skin and hair. Mixture of Vitamin A (retinol) palmate plus carotene, Vitamin A (retinol) palmitate plus fish oils and carotene (vegetable oils).

Danger of Using Alone: None known.

*This is a fat-soluble vitamin, which may build up in the body. Be careful not to exceed recommended dosage.

Vitamin B₁ — Thiamine

Natural Sources: Brewer's yeast, wheat germ, bran, liver, rice polishings, most whole grain cereals (especially wheat, oats, and rice), all seeds and nuts, beans (especially soy beans), milk and milk products, beets, potatoes, and leafy green vegetables.

Biochemical Uses: For the utilization of carbohydrates in energy production. Promotes healthy central nervous system, mental attitude. Helps prevent constipation, maintain normal red count, prevents edema and improves circulation.

Flagrant Clinical Symptoms: Beriberi, neuritis, edema.

Non-detectable Clinical Symptoms: Muscle cramps, weakness, slow heart beat, irritability, loss of appetite, fatigue, digestive disorders (including constipation), diabetes, depression, exhaustion.

RDA Requirements: 1.5 mg.

Supplement Amounts: 10 to 25 mg. daily, may go up to 100 mg. daily for limited periods.

Possible Help in Disease and Prevention: Aids in metabolism of carbohydrates, maintains nervous system, aids in protein metabolism. Prevents beriberi. Aids in breakdown of lactic acids which energize the body. Helps prevent constipation. Improves circulation. Stimulates appetite. Helps maintain normal blood count.

Toxicity: High dosage may cause irregular heartbeat in an occasional individual. If so, reduce dosage.

Synergistic Effect of this vitamin: For best result, B-complex should be administered simultaneously, otherwise singular use of any one of the B-vitamins can cause depletion of others in the body.

Danger of Using Alone: Prolonged ingestion of large doses of any of the B-complex vitamins alone may result in high urinary losses of other B-vitamins and lead to deficiencies.

Vitamin B₃ — Niacin

Natural Sources: Liver, brewer's yeast, kidney, wheat germ, whole grains, fish, eggs, lean meats, nuts, green vegetables, peanuts, sunflower seeds.

Biochemical Uses: Healthy brain functioning, nervous system, skin, circulation of the blood, protein and carbohydrate metabolism.

Flagrant Clinical Symptoms: Pellagra, neurasthenia, mental disease.

Vitamin B₂ — Riboflavin

Natural Sources: Milk, liver, enriched cereals, brewer's yeast, leafy green vegetables, fish, eggs, whole grains, wheat germs, almonds, sunflower seeds.

Biochemical Uses: Good vision, healthy skin, nails, and hair. Functions with other substances to breakdown and utilize carbohydrates, fats, and proteins.

Flagrant Clinical Symptoms: Ariboflavinosis (lesions of the mouth, lips, skin, and genitalia.)

Vitamin B₃ — Niacin

Non-detectable Clinical Symptoms: Nervousness, insomnia, canker sores, diarrhea, anemia, coated tongue, skin lesions, chronic headache.

RDA Requirements: 20 mg.

Supplement Amount: 50 - 100 mg. with meals daily

Possible Help in Disease and Prevention: Treatment of schizophrenia, pellagra, prevention of migraine headaches, improve circulation.

Toxicity: May cause stomach ulcers, liver damage, jaundice, colitis, and male impotence. In higher doses, some people may experience "niacin flush" which is a burning, prickly sensation. Those taking high blood pressure medication are particularly susceptible.

Synergistic Effects: See B₁

Danger of Using Alone: Take with all B-complex vitamins.

Vitamin B₂ — Riboflavin

Bloodshot eyes, abnormal sensitivity to light, itching and burning of the eyes, inflammations of the mouth, sore and burning tongue, cracks on the lips or corners of the mouth, dull or oily hair, excema, split nails. Can contribute to seborrhea, anemia, vaginal itching, cataracts, and ulcers.

1.7 mg.

10 to 25 mg. daily, may go up to 100 for limited periods.

In combination with Vitamin A, prevents and corrects cataracts, and improves health of skin and hair, general health and growth. Aids metabolism of carbohydrates, amino acids, and fatty acids. Helps body assimilate iron. Prevents premature wrinkles and split nails.

None Known

see B₁

Take with all B-complex vitamins.

Vitamin B₁₂ — Cobalamin

Natural Sources: Liver, dairy products, eggs, fortified brewer's yeast, sunflower seeds, comfrey leaves, kelp, bananas, peanuts, concord grapes, raw wheat germ, pollen.

Biochemical Uses: Maintenance of healthy nervous system, utilization of carbohydrates, fats, and proteins, regeneration of red blood cells, proper growth in children.

Flagrant Clinical Symptoms: Pernicious anemia, brain damage, degeneration of the nervous system.

Non-detectable Clinical Symptoms: Chronic fatigue, nervousness, heart palpitations, sore mouth and tongue, numbness or stiffness, difficulty in concentrating.

RDA Requirements: 3 mcg.

Supplement Amount: 1 to 5 mcg. Therapeutic doses of 50 to 100 mcg (usually injected). For vegetarians: take this vitamin naturally in the form of milk products, since vegetables contain only small amounts.

Possible Help in Disease and Prevention: Prevents anemia, prevents degeneration of the nervous system.

Toxicity: None known.

Synergistic Effects: Works with Folic Acid to cure pernicious anemia.

Danger of Using Alone: Always include other B-complex vitamins.

Vitamin B — Para-Aminobenzoic Acid (PABA)

Liver, kidney, whole grains, dairy products, eggs, wheat germ, molasses.

Helps in the formation of Folic Acid and the utilization of protein. Promotes growth, stimulates metabolism, healthy skin, protection against sun's burning rays.

Infertility, vitiligo, depression, excema, anemia, reproductive disorders.

Fatigue, headache, graying hair.

None established.

Up to 30 mg. without prescription. Higher dosages with prescription.

Prevents skin changes from aging process. Protection and prevention of sunburn and skin cancer.

Possible toxicity in high dosage.

None known.

Use with other B-complex vitamins.

Day 3 Eating For Your Health And Happiness

Vitamin B9 — Folic Acid

Natural Sources: Liver, leafy green vegetables, eggs, kidney, wheat germ, broccoli, asparagus, lima beans, Irish potatoes, mushrooms, nuts, brewer's yeast.

Biochemical Uses: Division of body cells and for the production of nucleic acids (RNA and DNA). For the utilization of sugar and amino acids.

Flagrant Clinical Symptoms: Pernicious anemia, megaloblastic anemia of pregnancy, serious skin disorders.

Non-detectable Clinical Symptoms: Fatigue, skin disorders, loss of libido in males, spontaneous abortion in females (miscarriage), impaired circulation, loss of hair.

RDA Requirement: 0.4 mg.

Supplement Amount: Up to 0.4 mg. is maximum allowed by F.D.A. Anything over 0.1 mg. available only by prescription and should be used only under medical doctor's supervision.

Possible Help in Disease and Prevention: Helps build antibodies to prevent and heal infections. Used for diarrhea, dropsy, stomach ulcers, menstrual problems, treatment of atherosclerosis, circulation problems, anemia, radiation injuries.

Toxicity: Possible toxicity in high dosage.

Synergistic Effects: None known.

Danger of Using Alone: When used without B_{12}, may mask symptoms of pernicious anemia.

Vitamin B — Inositol

Natural Sources: Liver, brewer's yeast, whole grains, wheat germ, unrefined molasses, corn, citrus fruits, lima beans, peas, organ meats, lecithin, nuts, milk.

Biochemical Uses: Combines with choline to form lecithin which metabolizes fat and cholesterol. Aids in hair growth. Promotes healthy heart muscle. Can reduce cholesterol level in blood.

Flagrant Clinical Symptoms: Exzema, high blood cholesterol.

Non-detectable Clinical Symptoms: Hair loss, constipation.

RDA Requirement: Does not recognize as essential.

Supplement Amount: 10 to 1,000 mg. daily (over 500 mg. considered therapeutic).

Possible Help in Disease and Prevention: Helps reduce blood cholesterol. In treatment of obesity and schizophrenia.

Toxicity: None known.

Synergistic Effects: None known.

Danger of Using Alone: Use with other B-complex vitamins.

Vitamin B — Choline

Natural Sources: Granular or liquid lecithin, brewer's yeast, wheat germ, egg yolk, leafy green vegetables, legumes, liver, kidney.

Biochemical Uses: Combines with inositol to form lecithin. Aids liver functions and kidneys, synthesis of nucleic acids. Minimizes excessive deposits of fat and cholesterol in liver and arteries, essential for myelin sheaths of the nerves. Prevention of gall stones, aids gall bladder function.

Flagrant Clinical Symptoms: Kidney damage, high blood pressure, cirrhosis, atherosclerosis, hardening of the arteries.

Non-detectable Clinical Symptoms: Deterioration of the kidneys, high blood pressure, fatty deterioration of the liver.

RDA Requirement: Not established.

Supplement Amount: 500 to 1,000 mg. daily (up to 3,000 plus for therapeutic purposes under medical doctor's supervision).

Possible Help in Disease and Prevention: Decrease amount of fat and cholesterol in liver and arteries. Used in treatment of nephritis. Provides protection against heart disease and stress.

Toxicity: None known.

Synergistic Effects: None known.

Danger of Using Alone: None known.

Vitamin B5 — Pantothenic Acid

Natural Sources: Whole grains, wheat germ, bran, kidney, liver, egg yolk, brewer's yeast, green vegetables, peas, beans, peanuts, molasses.

Biochemical Uses: Conversion of fat and sugar into energy. Effective utilization of PABA, choline, and fats. Maintains healthy nervous system and all vital functions of the body. Prevents infections. Helps in growth and regeneration.

Flagrant Clinical Symptoms: Hypoglycemia, duodenal ulcers, skin disorders, low blood pressure.

Non-detectable Clinical Symptoms: Restlessness, muscle cramps, burning sensation in feet, chronic fatigue, depression, retarded growth, allergies, asthma.

RDA Requirement: 10 mg.

Supplement Amount: 30 to 50 mg. (50 to 200 mg. considered therapeutic).

Possible Help in Disease and Prevention: Anti-stress factor. Prevents premature aging. Protects against effects of excessive radiation. Fights infections. Helps cure arthritis. May lower high blood pressure.

Toxicity: None known.

Synergistic Effects: None known.

Danger of Using Alone: Use with other B-complex vitamins.

Vitamin B₆ — Pyridoxine

Natural Sources: Brewer's yeast, wheat bran, rice bran, wheat germ, liver, kidney, heart, blackstrap molasses, milk, eggs, cabbage, beef, ham, lima beans, corn, pecans, green leafy vegetables.

Biochemical Uses: Metabolism of amino acids, building of blood, metabolism of fats, proteins & sugar, and normal functioning of the brain, nervous system, and muscles. Aids in production of antibodies, synthesis of RNA & DNA, regulation of sodium & potassium levels in the body.

Flagrant Clinical Symptoms: Anemia, blindness, peripheral neuropathy (both motor and sensory deficiencies in lower extremities), glossitis (sore mouth and lips), seborrhea, eczema, some drug-resistant convulsions in infants.

Non-detectable Clinical Symptoms: Loss of hair, water retention during pregnancy, nervousness, loss of appetite, diarrhea, anemia, depression, halitosis, degenerative diseases of old age.

RDA Requirement: 2 mg.

Supplement Amount: 10 to 25 mg. in divided doses several times a day.

Possible Help in Disease and Prevention: Produces antibodies to protect against bacterial invasions, prevents nervous and skin disorders, protects against degenerative diseases (such as high cholesterol and diabetes), prevents tooth decay and heart disease, lessens epileptic seizures, prevents pre-menstrual edema, is effective in treatment of Parkinson's Disease. Reduces oiliness of skin and acne, sensitivity to sun. Prevention of tooth decay. Natural diuretic.

Toxicity: None known. It may turn urine yellow, but is normal.

Synergistic Effects: None known.

Danger of Using Alone: Use with other B-complex vitamins.

Vitamin B₁₃** — Orotic Acid

Natural Sources: Whey portion of milk.

Biochemical Uses: Biosynthesis of nucleic acid, regenerative processes of cells.

Flagrant Clinical Symptoms: Overall degeneration as in multiple sclerosis. Cell degeneration.

Non-detectable Clinical Symptoms: Liver disorders, premature aging.

RDA Requirement: Not established.

Supplement Amount: Not known.

Possible Help in Disease and Prevention: Used in treatment of multiple sclerosis.

Toxicity: None known.

Synergistic Effects: None known.

Danger of Using Alone: None known.

Vitamin B**₁₅ — Pangamic Acid

**Although the proper name given is "vitamin" more appropriate would be the term "nutrient," since these have not been biochemically proven to be vitamins in a laboratory.

Natural Sources: Whole grains, seeds, nuts.

Biochemical Uses: Regulates fat metabolism. Stimulates glandular and nervous systems, increases body's tolerance to hypoxia (insufficient oxygen supply).

Flagrant Clinical Symptoms: Hypoxia, heart disease, glandular and nervous disorders.

Non-detectable Clinical Symptoms: Glandular and nervous disorders.

RDA Requirement: Not established.

Supplement Amount: 100 mg. daily.

Possible Help in Disease and Prevention: Increases body's tolerance to hypoxia. Used in treatment of heart disease, angina, high blood cholestarol, impaired circulation, and premature aging. Effective detoxicant.

Toxicity: None known.

Synergistic Effects: None.

Danger of Using Alone: None.

Biotin (Also called Vitamin H or Coenzyme R)

Natural Sources: Brewer's yeast, egg yolk, liver, milk, kidney, unpolished rice, soybeans. (Biotin is also produced in the intestines).

Biochemical Uses: Metabolism of proteins and fats, hair growth, used by thyroid and adrenal glands, reproductive tract, and nervous system.

Flagrant Clinical Symptoms: Dermatitis, depression, anemia, anorexia, eczema, seborrhea, pallor, heart abnormalities, hallucinations, lung infections.

Non-detectable Clinical Symptoms: Depression, peeling skin, loss of appetite, confusion, fatigue, dandruff, hair loss.

RDA Requirement: 0.3 mg.

Supplement Amount: 150 to 300 mcg.

Possible Help in Disease and Prevention: Treatment of malaria. Antiseptic. Prevents hair loss.

Toxicity: None known.

Synergistic Effects: None known.

Danger of Using Alone: Use with B-complex vitamins.

Day 3 Eating For Your Health And Happiness

Vitamin B**$_{17}$ — Nitrilosides (Laetrile)

Natural Sources: Most whole seeds of fruits, many grains, vegetables.

Biochemical Uses: Possible prevention and control of cancer.

Flagrant Clinical Symptoms: Malignancies (cancer)

Non-detectable Clinical Symptoms: None.

RDA Requirement: Not established.

Supplement Amount:

Possible Help in Disease and Prevention: Possible aid in prevention and control of cancer when taken with other supplement and total health program.

Toxicity: None known.

Synergistic Effect: None known.

Danger of Using Alone: Not known.

Vitamin C — Ascorbic Acid

All fresh fruits and vegetables. Particularly rich sources: rose hips, citrus fruits, black currants, strawberries, apples, persimmons, guavas, acerola cherries, potatoes, cabbage, broccoli, tomatoes, turnip greens, green bell peppers.

Essential for healthy condition of all bones and tissues, for proper functioning of adrenal and thyroid glands. Protects against all forms of stress, both physical and mental.

Bleeding and receding gums, unexplained bruises, slow healing, muscular weakness.

55 to 60 mg. daily

2000 mg. daily

Aids resistance to infections, formation of collagen (connective cement). Promotes healing. Prevents and cures common cold. Helps prevent stress reactions. Counteracts toxicity of drugs. Aids functioning of thyroid and adrenal glands. Has been used as a natural antibiotic.

Non-toxic. May sometimes have a laxative effect on some people. Although very rare, may precipitate formation of kidney stones in some sensitive people.

Helpful to take milk or calcium tablets. B_{12} is recommended along with this vitamin.

Vitamin D — Calciferol**

Natural Sources: Fish liver oil, milk and dairy products, sunlight, vegetables, sprouted seeds, mushroom, sunflower seeds.

Biochemical Uses: Essential for utilization of calcium and phosphorous. Necessary for strong teeth and bones, health of thyroid gland.

Flagrant Clinical Symptoms: Rickets, osteomalicia, retarded growth and poor bone formation in children, muscular weakness, lack of vigor, weight loss, loss of appetite.

Non-detectable Clinical Symptoms:

RDA Requirement: 400 I.U. daily. Therapeutically, up to 4,000 units a day for adults, half this for children, if not taken for more than one month.

Supplement Amount: 400 to 800 I.U. daily.

Possible Help in Disease and Prevention: Prevention of rickets. Helps prevent tooth decay and pyorrhea. Regulates absorbtion of calcium, phosphorous, and other minerals. Prevents skin diseases such as acne and psoriasis. Maintains normal basal metabolism, health of thyroid gland.

Toxicity: Can be toxic if taken in excessive doses.

Synergistic Effect: Best absorbed if taken with meals.

Danger of Using Alone: Prolonged ingestion may lead to renal (kidney) damage.

Vitamin F — Essential Fatty Acids**

Unrefined vegetable oils.

Normal glandular activity, healthy skin, mucous membranes. Promotes growth. Needed for many metabolic processes. Increases assimilation of calcium and phosphorous in the cells. Lowers blood cholesterol.

Skin disorders, eczema, acne, gall stones, reproductive disorders, kidney and prostate disorders.

Retarded growth, falling hair.

Not established.

Essential fatty acids at least 1% of total caloric intake of day (from National Research Council).

Helps lower blood cholesterol in atherosclerosis. Can protect from damage done by excessive radiation. Promotes healthy skin and mucous membranes.

None known.

None.

None.

**Although the proper name given is "vitamin" more appropriate would be the term "nutrient," since these have not been biochemically proven to be vitamins in a laboratory.

Vitamin E — Tocopherol*

Natural Sources:	Unrefined vegetable oils, all raw or sprouted seeds, nuts, grains, fresh wheat germ, leafy green vegetables, eggs.
Biochemical Uses:	Oxygenates the tissues, dilates blood vessels and improves circulation. Anti-thrombin and natural anti-coagulant. Protects lungs and other tissues from pollution. Vital to reproductive system. Retards aging process, prevents unsaturated fatty acids, sex hormones- and fat-soluble vitamins from being destroyed in the body by oxygen.
Flagrant Clinical Symptoms:	Degeneration of coronary system, pulmonary embolism, strokes, heart disease, anemia.
Non-detectable Clinical Symptoms:	Reproductive disorders, miscarriages, sterility, muscular disorders, testicle shrinking.
RDA Requirement:	15 I.U. daily
Supplement Amount:	200 to 400 I.U. daily
Possible Help in Disease and Prevention:	Dilates blood vessels and improves circulation, prevents scar tissue formation in burns. Anti-thrombin and anti-coagulant. Prevention and treatment of heart diseases, asthma, angina, pectoris, emphysema, leg ulcers, varicose veins, hypoglycemia. Prevention and treatment of reproductive disorders. Possibly slows aging process and prevents cancer.
Toxicity:	None known. People with hypertension should always consult physician before taking. Could increase blood pressure in some rare individuals.
Synergistic Effects:	Best absorbed with wheat germ oil. When taken with iron source, effect can be destroyed.
Danger of Using Alone:	None.

Vitamin K — Mendadione*

Natural Sources:	Kelp, green plants, soybean oil, egg yolks, milk, liver oats, rye, wheat. Also manufactured in the intestines.
Biochemical Uses:	Helps produce prothrombin which aids in blood clotting, normal liver functioning, anti-hemorraging, vitality, and longevity.
Flagrant Clinical Symptoms:	Hemorrhages
Non-detectable Clinical Symptoms:	Lowered vitality, premature aging.
RDA Requirement:	Not estblished.
Supplement Amount:	Not established.
Possible Help in Disease and Prevention:	Anti-hemorrhaging. Important to produce prothrombin, which aids in blood clotting.
Toxicity:	None.
Synergistic Effects:	None.
Danger of Using Alone:	None.

*This is a fat-soluble vitamin which may build up in the body. Be careful not to exceed recommended dosage.

Vitamin P — Bioflavonoids **

Natural Sources:	Citrus fruits, green peppers, grapes, apricots, strawberries, black currants, cherries, prunes, paprika juice.
Biochemical Uses:	Strengthens walls of capillaries, prevents capillary hemorrhaging and in an anticoagulant. Protects against destruction of Vitamin C by oxidation.
Flagrant Clinical Symptoms:	Capillary fragility.
Non-detectable Clinical Symptoms:	"Black and blue" marks on skin, pain in legs and joints, weakness of muscles.
RDA Requirement:	Not established.
Supplement Amount:	50 to 200 mg.
Possible Help in Disease and Prevention:	Strengthens capillary walls. Anticoagulant. May prevent strokes. Beneficial in hypertension, respiratory infections, hemorrhoids, varicose veins, hemorrhaging, bleeding gums, retinal hemorrhages, radiation sickness, coronary thrombosis, artherosclerosis.
Toxicity:	None known.
Synergistic Effects:	Enhances properties of Vitamin C. Protects this vitamin from destruction in body by oxidation.
Danger of Using Alone:	None.

**Although the proper name given is "vitamin" more appropriate would be the term "nutrient," since these have not been biochemically proven to be vitamins in a laboratory.

Vitamin T** — "Sesame Seed Factor"

Natural Sources:	Sesame seeds, egg yolks, some vegetable oils.
Biochemical Uses:	Promotes formation of blood platelets, improves fading memory.
Possible Help in Disease and Prevention:	Re-established platelet integrity of blood. Corrects nutritional anemia.

Vitamin F** — "Flaxseed"

Natural Sources:	Flaxseed.
Biochemical Uses:	Helps body assimilate calcium.

**Although the proper name given is "vitamin" more appropriate would be the term "nutrient," since these have not been biochemically proven to be vitamins in a laboratory.

The importance of minerals and many of the trace minerals is becoming more relevant. It was a subject long left ignored in modern medicine, but now that our soils are so very depleted, the products grown in them are also depleted of these life-sustaining elements. It is time to begin paying more attention to the minerals in our diets.[24]

Mineral Guide

	Calcium	Phosphorous
Natural Sources:	Cheese, milk, grains such as oats, beans, almonds, walnuts, dark leafy green vegetables, especially the cabbage family, lettuce, endive.	Dairy products, eggs, fish, legumes, whole grains, seeds, nuts.
Functions:	Has role in basically all vital body functions. Helps maintain acid/alkaline balance of the body needed for muscle activity and regular heart beat. Essential for appropriate utilization of phosphorous, and vitamins A, D, and C. Important role in pregnancy and lactation. Needed for building teeth, bones, and normal growth development and cell division.	Necessary for healthy bones, teeth, and muscles. Needed for proper assimilation of fats and proteins. Essential for digestion of the B vitamins niacin and riboflavin. Helps body handle carbohydrates. Like magnesium, it is closely related to calcium and the two must be in proper balance.
RDA Requirement:	Adults—800 mg. daily. Children and pregnant and lactating women—1,000 to 1,400 mg. daily.	Adults—800 mg. daily Children and pregnant women—1,000 to 1,400 mg. daily
Supplement Amount:	Bone meal and calcium lactate are good natural supplements. Calcium lactate—3 to 5 tablets at bedtime. Bone Meal—1 gr. daily in divided doses.	100 to 500 mg. daily****

****White refined sugar disturbs the calcium/phosphorous balance resulting in arthritis. (From *The Complete Book of Minerals for Health*, J. I. Rodale and Staff, Rodale Books, Inc., Emmaus, PA, 1976.)

---

[24]*The Washington Post*, "The Small Elements of Good Eating," January 19, 1978.

MANGANESE

Natural Sources: Bran, peas and beans, kelp, wheat germ, green leafy vegetables, oatmeal, rye, citrus fruits.

Functions: Helps in digestion of utilization of fats. Necessary for normal reproduction. Very important to muscles, maternal emotion, and metabolism. (Sometimes called "The Big M")

RDA Requirement: Not known.

Supplement Amount: Taking bone meal as mentioned. This has manganese, calcium, and phosphorous.

MAGNESIUM

Natural Sources: Nuts, almonds, peanuts, whole grains, green leafy vegetables, apples, peaches, lemons, seeds (sesame and sunflower), brown rice.

Functions: Important in many enzyme reactions, especially connected with energy needed for maintenance of proper calcium and potassium levels in body and prevention of kidney damage. Essential for healthy heart, utilization of fats, vitamins E and B, and synthesis of proteins. Important in maintaining healthy nerves and muscles.

RDA Requirement: 350 mg. daily

Supplement Amount: 100 to 300 mg. daily

Natural Sources: Eggs, onions, brewer's yeast, garlic, tuna, milk, whole grains, kelp, seafood, mushrooms, vegetables grown in mineral-rich soils.

Function: An antioxidant effect similar to Vitamin E. Reduces free radicals. Helps protect against cancer through this action and perhaps reduce aging process. Helps regenerate damaged liver.

RDA Requirement: Not established.

Supplement Amount: 50 to 100 mcg. daily.

Toxicity: Can be toxic in high dosage, so be certain to follow instructions. Try to obtain selenium from organically grown foods.

Iron* + +

Natural Sources: Blackstrap molasses, brewer's yeast, kelp, whole grains and seeds (sun flower and sesame), beans, lentils, liver, egg yolks, peaches, raisins, prunes, bananas, apricots.

Function: Essential in the formation of hemoglobin which is the oxygen carrier. May increase resistance to disease and stress.

RDA Requirements: Males—10 mg. daily, Females—18 mg. daily.

Supplement Amount: 10 to 15 mg. daily

*+ +Coffee and tea interfere with absorption of iron.

Manganese

Magnesium

Selenium

Chromium ***

Whole grain bread, liver, mushrooms, brewer's yeast, hard mineralized water (depending on location).

Helps metabolism of sugars and starches. Works with insulin to improve insulin balance in blood. Plays role in serum cholesterol metabolism. Important integral part of many hormones and enzymes.

Not established.

Take as component of brewer's yeast.

Zinc* +

Seafoods, leafy green vegetables, grains and seeds (sprouted or fermented in sour dough), brewer's yeast, onions, milk, eggs.

Essential in many enzymatic processes and hormone activities, especially reproduction. Involved in carbohydrate metabolism necessary for formation of DNA and RNA and the synthesis of protein.

15 mg. daily

50 to 100 mg. daily. If under doctor's supervision, may be taken up to 500 mg. daily, as in aiding the healing process of wounds.

*****Refined white sugar depletes the body of Chromium.

* +Alcohol flushes zinc from the system, causing deficiency.

Iodine

Kelp, sea salt, parakelp, seaweed, citrus fruits, garlic, seafoods, fish liver oils, pineapple, pears, artichokes.

Essential for synthesis of thyroid hormone (thyroxin) which regulates much of our mental and physical activity. Regulates body metabolism and energy production. Necessary for health of thyroid gland.* + + +

.15 mg.

.1 to .2 mg. daily

*+ + +A fascinating and enlightening discussion of the importance of thyroid is presented in the book, *Hypothyroidism: The Unsuspected Illness*, by Broda A. Barnes, M.D., and Lawrence Galton, Thomas Y. Crowell Co., New York: 1976.

The Three Inexpensive Ways to Better Health

Although the taking of vitamin and mineral supplements is highly recommended for optimum health, there are three steps you can take that are inexpensive and very effective in achieving better health. These are:

1. Eliminate all refined sugar from your diet.
2. Eat whole grains every day (in the form of cereals and breads). You can buy an inexpensive seed and nut mill (grinder) for less than $10.00 and purchase your whole grains in bulk, grinding them yourself as needed.
3. Make sure that the water you are drinking is pure. For a further discussion of this topic, see the section entitled "Water—A Frightening Awakening" which follows.

Vitamin Toxicity

If you are concerned about vitamin toxicity, you might want to keep the following guidelines in mind. Basically, there are two types of vitamins: water-soluble and fat-soluble. The fat-soluble ones are D, E, A, and K. These are the ones that you should not take in great quantities, since they can remain in your body. The other vitamins are water-soluble, and remain for only a short time. This is why your doctor may tell you that you are wasting your money taking Vitamin C, since it can be washed out of your system. However, you may be retaining more than your doctor knows about. Personally, I would rather be on the side of taking a little more and perhaps losing some, than not taking enough.

Resistance from your doctor stems from the newness of the subject. Everything negative the doctors might tell you, I myself have said as many times in the past, before I really knew much about the subject. But through learning about supplements on my own and through nutritional courses, I now firmly believe that it is more sensible to chance losing some of the supplements than to have a deficiency in any of them. The pioneers and researchers in the area of nutrition deserve tremendous credit for their perserverance and discoveries. Acceptance of such discoveries takes time, but the news media (such as the Washington Post) deserve our thanks in their coverage of these crucial issues.

156 Total Glow

Water - A Frightening Awakening

In August of 1970, the Federal Government released a little-publicized report that sent chills up the spines of the people who had access to it. This report, and the warnings of Dr. Athelstan, a scientist at the University of Minnesota, are reason enough to make you think carefully about your water supply.

Some of the findings from these federal water experts reveal that there is a forty percent chance that the next glass of water you drink will have gone through an industrial conduit filled with chemical poisons, bacteria, waste, and sewerage. You may think that your water is being treated to remove the harmful wastes, but the degree of waste materials and poisons is becoming so great that the amount of chlorine added to treat the waste is resulting in carcinogenic by-products itself.

The National Cancer Institute director recognizes this problem and says, "We support the judgment that these chemicals present a potential risk of cancer that should be reduced to the extent feasible."

The fact remains that one out of four cities in this country depends upon drinking water that does not meet government standards.[25]

How Does Your City Rate in Safe Water?

The following chart comes from the Environmental Protection Agency, relating parts per billion of the chemical pollution in water supply in 113 cities. Under 100 ppb is considered safe.

1. Albuquerque, NM	15 ppb	16. Camden, AZ		120
2. Amarillo, TX	130	17. Cape Girardeau, MO		140
3. Annadale, VA	200	18. Casper, WY		41
4. Atlanta, GA	75	19. Charleston, SC		200
5. Baltimore, MD	65	20. Charlotte, NC		71
6. Baton Rouge, LA	1.6	21. Chattanooga, TN		98
7. Billings, MT	13	22. Cheyenne, WY		130
8. Birmingham, AL	75	23. Chicago, IL		50
9. Bismarck, ND	100	24. Cleveland, OH		49
10. Boise, ID	16	25. Columbus, OH		210
11. Boston, MA	5	26. Concord, CA		110
12. Brownsville, TX	450	27. Corvallis, OR		57
13. Buffalo, NY	23	28. Dallas, TX		79
14. Burlington, VT	91	29. Davenport, IO		100
15. California Aqueduct, CA	110	30. Dayton, OH		40
		31. Denver, CO		39

[25]*The National Health Federation Bulletin*, 1970, and *The Wall Street Journal*, June 13, 1978.

Day 3 Eating For Your Health And Happiness

32. Des Moines, IO	15	73. Oklahoma Cty, OK	200
33. Detroit, MI	34	74. Omaha, NE	120
34. Duluth, MN	12	75. Passiac Vly, NJ	130
35. Elizabeth, NJ	86	76. Phoenix, AZ	130
36. Erie, PA	31	77. Portland, ME	7.4
37. Eugene, OR	25	78. Portland, OR	20
38. Ft. Worth, TX	61	79. Poughkeepsie, NY	78
39. Ft. Wayne, IN	59	80. Providence, RI	8
40. Fresno, CA	0.37	81. Provo, UT	12
41. Grand Rapids, MI	69	82. Pueblo, CO	9.6
42. Greenville, MS	2.4	83. Richmond, VA	34
43. Hackensack, NJ	110	84. Rockford, IL	7.9
44. Hagerstown, MD	100	85. Rome, GA	79
45. Hartford, CT	36	86. Sacramento, CA	29
46. Houston, TX	250	87. St. Croix, Vir. Is.	23
47. Huntington, WV	110	88. St. Louis, MO	51
48. Huron, SD	300	89. St. Paul, MI	90
49. Illwaco, WA	250	90. Salt Lake City, UT.	43
50. Indianapolis, IN	82	91. San Antonio, TX	13
51. Jackson, MS	240	92. San Diego, CA	97
52. Jacksonville, FL	8.7	93. San Francisco, CA	78
53. Jersey City, NJ	64	94. Sante Fe, NM	180
54. Kansas City, MO	34	95. Sioux Falls, SD	79
55. Lincoln, NE	28	96. So. Pittsburgh, PA	43
56. Little Rock, AR	42	97. Spokane, WA	1.9
57. Los Angeles, CA	49	98. Springfield, MA	20
58. Las Vegas, NV	76	99. Syracuse, NY	18
59. Louisville, KY	150	100. Tacoma, WA	8.9
60. Madison, WI	0.02	101. Tampa, FL	230
61. Manchester, NH	60	102. Terrebonne Parish, LA	140
62. Melbourne, FL	550	103. Toledo, OH	38
63. Memphis, TN	17	104. Topeka, KA	180
64. Milwaukee, WI	16	105. Tulsa, OK	50
65. Monroe, MI	58	106. Washington, DC	110
66. Montgomery, AL	110	107. Waterbury, CT	110
67. Mt. Clemens, MI	48	108. Waterford Twnshp. NY	83
68. Nashville, TN	24	109. Wheeling, WV	160
69. New Haven, CT	49	110. Whiting, IN	3.6
70. Newport, RI	160	111. Wichita, KA	27
71. Norfolk, VA	150	112. Wilmington/Stanton DE	64
72. Oakland, CA	45	113. Yuma, AZ	86

Some Predictions and Alternatives

The chemicals primarily involved in this "purification" of water are trihalomethanes. These are formed when chlorine is added to water to kill bacteria and other organic chemicals introduced into the drinking water through pollution from rivers and ground water.

A thorough and well-studied work investigating these pollutants has been performed by International Publishers, written by Pierre Roridiere, along with a staff of international contributors. You can again witness the damage that is being done to our essential natural resources, ranging from DDT to detergents in our water supply. Remember that the human adult is comprised of approximately seventy-five pints of water. Do you want pollutants and possible carcinogens floating around throughout all those seventy-five pints?

Frightening enough is the evidence that our water is polluted, but now consider the fact that we are running *short* of water that humans can safely consume.[26]

Basing the calculations on the rate of consumption which will have been achieved in the United States between now and then, (1,950 cubic yards per year, per American) and setting this figure against the 15 thousand million population forecast by demographers for the year 2,030, after the end of that year, not one extra human being will be able to be supported unless something is done about the situation now.

"Those who foretell the future assert that unless vigorous communal action is taken on a global scale, catastrophies will be widespread after the year 2,010 (thirty years from now) and by 2,050, man will have been wiped out of Earth."[27] These estimates are conservative.

The Subject of Nitrates and Nitrites

Nitrosamines are the responsible carcinogens. However, they are formed from the action of nitrite. Nitrite, added to foods, then becomes the offender in producing diseases in our bodies. Nitrite, however, is produced by nitrate through microbial action, both inside and outside the body. Therefore, foods containing either substance lead to high levels of nitrite.

To discuss the biochemical reactions whereby this occurs is not relevant to the scope of this book. What is important is that most

---

[26] James Claude Wright, *The Coming Water Famine* (New York: Coward McCann, 1966).

[27] *Purity or Pollution — The Struggle for Water*, Pierre Rondiere. International Library, Collins Publishers, New York: 1971.

biochemists in the field agree about the dangers of nitrite/nitrate. The area of disagreement is the level at which these substances become dangerous. Don't depend on some outside authority to determine what is too high, start avoiding them right away. This applies to all substances which have not yet been proven safe for human consumption. Each one of us must look at what is beginning to appear in our water and food supplies. Even major newspapers are printing news to the effect that the level of chloroform is carcinogenic in our supplies, yet we are subjected to drinking it.

To get away from the nitrate/nitrite situation, purchase your sandwich meats and all-beef hot dogs in health food stores. They also offer sausage and salami which is fresh and without preservatives. These are clearly labeled "Without Nitrites or Nitrates." Try to patronize manufacturers of these products so that eventually the larger food companies will get the message.

Pet Nutrition

It is my contention that many people feed their pets better than themselves. We don't indulge them daily with refined sugar, sweets such as cake, pie, cookies, etc., nor do we give them overly-cooked vegetables or processed TV dinners. We leave these things to ourselves.

However, our pets are like us in many respects. Basically, they fall ill to most of the same diseases we do, and cancer is probably on the increase in the pet world, too.

Basic animal health requires a supply of the general nutrients humans need. Use a good dry food and read the labels well for additives and preservatives. Choose a brand low in these menaces.

Feed your pet a larger meal earlier in the day and make the evening feeding a light one. Don't send them out to exercise too soon after eating. This will impair their digestion and assimilation of their food.

Let your pets eat from your diet as a supplement. Our cat and dog eat essentially everything that we eat (including raw cabbage salad!). Some animals won't take seasoned foods right away, especially vegetables, but if you don't give in to their whims and continue to offer them these foods, they will soon develop a taste for nutritious leftovers and scraps. They will probably still prefer their own cat or dog food, but introduce them to table scraps from your own healthy diet.

Exercise your pets well about two hours after a main meal. If they are alone for long periods of time, quiet music is sometimes relaxing and calming. Let them listen to your radio while you're out of the house from time to time.

Supplementing a Pet's Diet:

Bone Meal: Contains a balance of calcium, magnesium phosphorous, and other important trace minerals. 1 to 2 teaspoons per day for a large dog, diminishing according to size and weight of dog. One half teaspoon per day for cats.

Liver pills: 1 to 4 tablets per day, according to pet size. You won't have any trouble getting your pet to accept these pills. My cat will pursue anything to get them.

Eggs: 2 eggs per week, raw or lightly boiled. Serve alone or mixed with other food.

Multiple vitamins: 1 tablet or capsule per day.

Lecithin: Sprinkle on food daily.

Oil: Several drops of safflower or sesame oil on food daily. May have a laxative effect in the beginning, but as your pet's diet changes, the oil will effectively balance out the fat content in the body.

Remember that exercise for your pet is as crucial as it is for you. Your dog will enjoy jogging or walking with you, so don't forget to take him/her along on your exercise jaunts. Some cats can be trained to a collar and leash, and yours might enjoy a walk around the neighborhood in this manner.

Day 4
Implementing The Plan

SUGGESTIONS FOR ACHIEVING TOTAL GLOW

Now that you have gained a rather intensive introduction to the Total Glow program and what it entails, you might be asking yourself, "How can I get all of this to apply to me and my life?"

Certainly there will be some elements or areas that will not appeal to you or that cannot be incorporated into your lifestyle, and other areas in which you feel no great need to improve. It is to be strongly emphasized, however, that improvement in any one of these areas will be greatly enhanced and expedited by similar improvement in the other two areas.

Everyone wants to improve their health, their appearance, and their personal interactions in the world. The benefits will be life-long, and will touch every facet of your life. It is a current opinion in various media that thinner businesspeople have a far greater chance of advancement, and that they earn higher salaries than do those who are more portly. No one needs to tell you that someone with a healthy, pleasant outlook on life is going to be more fun to be around and easier to work with. Possessing the poise, fitness, and self-confidence that health and optimum muscle tone engenders will carry you through many rough spots, simply because you will be feeling good about yourself.

Some further suggestions that might help carry you through the Total Glow program would be:

1. Start gradually. While I'm not promoting overnight miracles, I will tell you that you will feel better very soon. There is then a tendency to rush into the program full force. If you rush, it's easier for you to drop out or feel as if you are failing in some respect. Don't be in a hurry. You'll feel the benefits soon enough,

and you'll be feeling better (at leat psychologically) every day that you're on the program. Some people who are sicker than they realize may not feel as good as quickly. Be patient. It took years to deplete your body, and overnight recovery isn't an appropriate expectation.

2. Visit a health food store (or "natural food" store) in your area. Look around, ask questions, sample the products. Remember that healthful food without additives may taste differently initially because your palate has been conditioned to the taste of the additives in most processed foods. Give yourself time to develop a taste for these pure foods. Like fine wine and blue cheese, they are something quite delicious, but you need to get used to them.

There has been a great deal of controversy lately about the value of products sold in health food stores. Some sources report that the only difference between these products as opposed to ordinary supermarket food is that the health food is twice as expensive. Happily, many supermarkets are beginning to stock preservative-free foods. Once you get used to recognizing the brands, you might find it easier to locate these items in your local supermarket. Consistent use of them will cause your grocer to stock more of them. If not, ask that they be stocked.

In matters of expense, think about your health. The argument about higher prices is quite specious to say the least. Compare the cost of eating dinner in a fast food restaurant three times a week to buying purer food and eating at home. Your budget will be the guide, and better health the result.

3. You might consider enrolling in an exercise class. These programs are offered quite inexpensively through you local YMCA's or YWCA's or through Adult Education Departments of area schools and colleges. If you really want to pamper yourself, consider enrolling in an organized program at a health spa or fitness center. Use caution, however, and thoroughly investigate the facility before signing any contract. Many so-called figure salons are merely expensive calisthenics classes lead by an inexperienced or unqualified teacher. You might get just as good a workout at the local "Y" or in a nearby high school gym, for a quarter of the price.

At the spa or center, investigate the equipment and services to which you will have access, ask to meet your instructors, and find out about their credentials. Determine whether or not the spa will tailor-make a special program suited to your needs, and take a look at the showers, the sauna, massage rooms, pool, and locker room areas to make sure they are satisfactory.

4. Make an appointment with your physician. Tell him or her that you are planning to embark upon a self-improvement program which will include relaxation, exercise, and nutrition. Your doctor will be able to advise you if there are any special requirements or areas that need special attention. Also, the doctor will be aware of your efforts and will be better prepared to measure your progress and foresee any difficulties.

5. Make it a point to THINK EXERCISE as often and as much as possible. Try to break out of your sedentary lifestyle. Take the stairs. Get out and do some brisk walking. Stop letting yourself be chauffered around. Do your errands yourself. Set aside a certain time each day to do some at-desk or at-home exercises.

6. Decide that you are going to cut down in the junk foods in your diet. Contrary to popular opinion, there are literally thousands of foods that are not only delicious, but are healthful and non-fattening. Instead of indulging in heavy, fattening martini lunches, pack a low-calorie lunch and eat at your desk. But always try to get in a brisk walk sometime during the day, and come back via the stairs.

Instead of the usual snacks, take a small plastic bag filled with carrots and celery sticks. If you place an ice cube inside the bag and tie it securely, your raw vegetables will stay chilled and crisp until lunch time. This is also great for cocktail food or appetizers. Serve a platter filled with carrots, celery, cauliflower, radishes, raw squash, and raw spinach. Offer a dip or two from the recipes in this book. A loaf of freshly-baked rye bread on the table would be a delicious and inviting accompaniment. Try to serve as many raw and fresh snacks as possible.

The following is the Total Glow Health Policy, which you might want to tape up on the wall where you will see it often:

The Total Glow Health Policy

Drink pure water. Have it tested.

Learn to relax in any type of situation.

Develop an exercise program that best suits you.

Buy only vegetables and fruits that are free from sprays, chemicals, and insecticides.

Give yourself appropriate sleep and rest each day.

Buy only meat, fish, and poultry that has not been exposed to or fed harmful chemicals.

Eliminate refined sugar from you diet.

Increase the level of raw foods in your diet.

Read labels on every can, bottle, and package, and avoid all chemicals, additives, dyes, artificial flavors and colors as much as possible.

Decrease your salt intake by substituting herbs and spices.

Don't get angry and punish yourself for any setbacks or regressions you might make. These are normal.

Say to yourself, "I will forgive myself when I make a mistake. To err is human, but to forgive myself is so difficult that it is divine."

Admit your mistakes.

Accept praise and compliments.

LISTEN to what other people are saying. This is the best way to learn about yourself, your world, and the people you care about.

Special Considerations: The Popcorn Problem

Keeping these simple guidelines in mind will make the road to a more relaxed, healthy, and vital life easier and more enjoyable. At the same time, you shouldn't feel guilty or try to punish yourself for an occasional "transgression." In fact, it might be better for you to institute some kind of built-in reward or "treat" system so that it can reinforce your progress.

Let's take an example. One follower of the Total Glow program explained that she thoroughly enjoyed the program and found it exceptionally quick in producing results. There was one problem, however, that really bothered her and she asked for further advice.

She explained that her weakness was popcorn. She was able to avoid all other junk foods but that one, and no matter how hard she tried to substitute raw vegetables, dried fruits and nuts, or something else, she found it impossible to stay away from popcorn. So whenever she did have popcorn, she made herself feel guilty, as if all her good work had been un-done. Then it was even harder for her to get back into proper eating and exercising because she felt so badly about not maintaining her new healthy lifestyle.

This kind of experience is so common that I would be remiss in failing to mention it. But unlike most diets, this one allows for an occasional indulgence of favorite treats.

The solution to her problem was quite simple. She can eat popcorn! Of course it is not to be concluded that you may eat popcorn until you are sick and that it won't harm you. The fact is that she loved popcorn, and to deprive her of that would have been destructive to her program. It would have been setting her up against an authority figure. Besides, popcorn can be healthy.

I recommended that she visit a health food store and locate some natural, organic popcorn which she could make for herself. When she did cook popcorn, it was advised that she make a smaller quantity and put it in a smaller bowl. After the popcorn was popped, and before eating it, she should wash out the popper and put it away. These actions would effectively prevent her from overindulging and give her the impression that she had had all that she wanted.

Incidentally, popcorn is a food that is naturally high in fiber and can be very good for you. In fact, due to its nutritional content, it is probably one of the best snacks available. Just watch that you don't over-salt it or eat it too often, as with any other food.

The Hot Fudge Sundae Solution

Perhaps there is a special treat you really enjoy that does not offer such a simple solution. Here is an example from another follower of my Total Glow program:

"My weakness is chocolate fudge sundaes. I can't live without chocolate fudge sundaes, and I usually have one every night for dessert. What can I do about this? Is there a way I can make sundaes healthier and less fattening?"

This one is somewhat harder to solve than the popcorn situation, but there is a solution. First, try to cut down on the frequency. Tell yourself that you are going to change your destructive eating habits. If, on occasion, you really want something, then have it and don't feel guilty. But don't overdo it as you have in the past.

Replace the ice cream with frozen yogurt. Yogurt is a delicious natural snack which has received a great deal of attention from the media. Whether or not the advertising claims are one hundred percent truthful or not, natural yogurt does contain a bacteria which interacts beneficially in the digestive system. It is also lower in fat and sugars than regular ice cream, and has fewer calories, preservatives, and additives. Look for 100% natural yogurt sweetened with honey rather than refined sugar, make your own yogurt, or use natural honey ice cream without preservatives, such as Haagen Daaz.

Next, you can figure out a way to make your own chocolate fudge sauce that will not be as sugar-saturated or have as many chemicals as the brand from the supermarket. Read the label on that jar and ask yourself if you honestly want to put all those chemicals into your body. There is a recipe for chocolate fudge sauce in the recipe section, and it is made with carob chips rather than chocolate.

Carob is a root that tastes surprisingly like chocolate and can be used as a healthy substitute for just about any recipe calling for chocolate. A fellow writer once owned a chain of candy stores and he was a self-admitted chocolate "addict." But when he tried the carob fudge, he switched. Now, if a person who makes his own chocolate candies and fudge can like carob fudge enough to swear off the other kind, it's got to be good enough for you! In the recipe, use only natural ingredients and flavorings. Sprinkle the top with a mixture of freshly shredded coconut and crushed or roasted nuts.

See how easy that is? Now you have a complete chocolate fudge sundae that you will be able to enjoy more, knowing that it is healthier for you than the other kind since it is totally without harmful additives and chemicals.

These examples are used to illustrate a basic concept; there ARE methods that can be successfully employed in order to bypass less beneficial habits. With a little imagination, you will be able to come up with these solutions yourself. A handy reference tool would be this book in conjunction with a regular cookbook. When you want to make something, first look up the recipe in the ordinary cookbook, then refer to this one for hints on cutting calories, using more natural ingredients, or substituting healthful foods for harmful ones.

The following steps are some suggestions for beginning your own individual program.

GUIDELINES—How To Do It

Gradual Approach

Take your time. There are many people who are anxious to plunge head-first into any new experience, who will rampage their kitchen, throwing out every can and package that lists something unhealthy on the label. If you are that kind of person, go ahead and get involved 100% right away, but don't get discouraged. Don't set yourself up for a fall.

I would recommend that you proceed slowly, and gradually acquire healthy items for your kitchen. Particularly if your interest in healthful foods meets with even the slightest resistance from your family, I would suggest that you proceed with extra care. Try to put yourself in your family's place and empathize with their possible feelings of your infringement on their rights. After all, they are used to their diets and chances are that they like what they have been eating. Your suddenly telling them that it is "bad" will set you up as that authority figure against whom to rebel!

It has taken you some time to become convinced of the value of healthful eating. Give those around you the same amount of time to warm up to the subject.

Fresh Fruits

Begin offering fresh fruits as snacks and desserts. In the summertime, when strawberries, blueberries, blackberries, and raspberries are plentiful, plan on freezing big batches so that you may enjoy these delicious fruits all year 'round. Whenever you can, stock up on apples, peaches, bananas, fresh pineapple, pears, oranges, and grapefruit. If you continually have fresh fruit around the house, you are more likely to prefer it over a period of time to the more sticky-sweet or salty snacks. A great dessert to follow a big meal would be a compote of orange and grapefruit sections, chunks of fresh pineapple, banana slices, and raisins, topped off with shredded coconut and a dollop of honey-sweetened yogurt. You can also mix strawberries, and the different kinds of melon quite successfully.

Try to get away from using canned fruits, unless you can find the water-pack variety. Even so, these have been heated to the extent that they are not as nutritious as fresh. If your family likes gelatin desserts and salads, you might switch to the dietetic kind. Very few people can detect the difference when fruit or vegetables are added. Use shredded carrots, cabbage, and water-pack fruits, and adapt your current gelatin recipes to more low-calorie dishes. Remember, though, that even diet gelatins contain artificial colors and preservatives, so try to break away from all flavored gelatins gradually and substitute plain gelatin, adding your own flavors.

Dried Fruits

Next to fresh fruits, dried fruits are the most nutritious, especially if they are organically grown and are free from preservatives and additives. These dried fruits (such as apples, apricots, dates, pineapple, figs, and prunes) are delicious and store well in the refrigerator. You can mix them with raw nuts, seeds, and cereal for a really satisfying snack. When visiting a health food store, ask to sample their offerings of dried fruit/nut snack mixes. Chances are that you can figure out how to make your own by noting the ingredients. Small shops offering raw and freshly roasted nuts are fast growing in popularity in America, and you can buy your nuts, seeds, and dried fruits from them.

New Experiences With Bread

On your next trip to the grocery store, try skipping the white bread and select one or two whole grain substitutes. This is probably the one area where you will meet the least resistance from your family, since these breads actually taste much better than supermarket bread. If you seem to meet with reluctance, you can at least serve a darker bread every other day until they develop a preference for whole-grain breads. If you have the time, experiment with the bread recipes offered in this book. There really isn't anything more inviting than the smell of freshly baked bread emanating from your kitchen. Your family might just come running! The hardest thing about baking bread is having enough time to do it. There is a recipe for no-knead bread included.

Yogurt

If you use a great deal of sour cream, an ideal substitute is unflavored natural yogurt. This can go in many salads, dips, dressings, soups, and meat dishes. Next time someone asks you what you'd like for your birthday, you might consider suggesting a yogurt maker. These are relatively inexpensive items, use very little electricity, and are almost fail-proof. Yogurt makers are especially nice because you have a constant supply on hand and do not have to remember to buy sour cream whenever you need it in a recipe. Unlike sour cream, yogurt is naturally low in calories, and contains a valuable enzyme that aids in digestion.

The Natural Food Dinner Party

Socially, you might consider getting together with a few friends who share your interest in healthful eating and have a totally natural food dinner party. A Party Buffet Menu Plan is included in this book. The recipes that you can come up with should be intriguing, and it might be a good way to introduce reluctant spouses to the many epicurean pleasures of natural foods.

Fruits and Vegetables

Fruit and vegetable juices are another easy area in which to make the transition. Although more and more companies are offering preservative- and additive-free juices on the supermarket shelves, it is still quite simple to make your own or at least start sampling them in health food stores. Do this gradually at first. Some juices are quite strongly flavored, especially for a palate that is accustomed to preservatives. If you try one that you feel is overpowering, you can dilute it with one half water, or some other juice. Carrot juice in particular is strong for most people who are just beginning to sample natural juices. Try mixing it first with water and then mixing it with V8 or tomato juice. If you have a blender, you can add all kinds of delicious vegetables to plain tomato juice, such as celery, carrots, cabbage, beets, and radishes. Diluting with water not only reduces the sweetness of the fruit juices, but decreases the cost and calories.

Another very special treat your family is certain to enjoy is freshly squeezed citrus juice. Try surprising them with a nice glass of fresh, chilled orange or grapefruit juice next Saturday morning. This is the best way to introduce natural juices, since most everybody loves citrus juice.

Try to offer your family healthy fruit and vegetable juices in place of soft drinks or canned fruit "drinks." Soft drinks are 100% refined sugar, artificial flavorings, artificial colorings, and chemically bombarded water. Fruit "drinks" that come in large cans are almost wholly refined sugar, artificial colorings, artificial flavorings, with a minute amount of redeeming Vitamin C thrown in, almost as an afterthought. Even so, the Vitamin C is synthetic, and the heating process necessary for canning destroys much of it. The canned drinks aren't much better for you than the powdered kind that comes in an envelope to which you add your own sugar. Much of it is artificial. You can certainly do without them, and natural fruit juices taste incomparably better.

Coffee Substitutes

Coffee drinking is an area where you might wish to taper off gradually. The instant varieties with preservatives are not healthy, so you might start by making your coffee from ground beans. Take a thermos of freshly made ground coffee to work with you rather than a jar of instant. You might also consider grinding your own and freezing it so that it remains fresh. If this isn't possible, there are a few new brands of instant coffee that are totally natural and without preservatives. Read the labels before you buy.

One such instant coffee was discovered recently by an associate. It is advertised as an "instant coffee and grain beverage" by the name of Mellow Roast™ and contains coffee, bran, wheat, and molasses. In addition to being mellower and less bitter than regular instant coffee, it has a pleasant wheaty flavor. This is available in your supermarket. In health food stores, look for a similar product called Pero.™

Another method of kicking the "coffee habit" (if you have one) would be to start sampling herb teas. Sometimes you can buy what is called a "sampler" of herb teas that contain one or more bags of an assortment of teas. These are delicious and have been found to aid digestion, quiet the stomach, and soothe jangled nerves. Again, as with fruit and vegetable juices, you may not like all of them. Try several kinds and use the ones you like. They come in flavors like peppermint, rosehip, camomile, red zinger, spearmint, rostarma, and comfrey leaf.

Brown Rice

In the same way that refined sugar has lost all its nutrients in processing, so has rice. When rice is polished, the outer coverings are removed. The rice is then heated and bleached, robbing it of its beneficial nutrients. What is left, after 90% of the food value has been removed is then "enriched" with synthetic vitamins and minerals. These, too, are usually lost in the cooking process.

As an alternative, use brown rice. This is high in Vitamin B-complex since the outer layers have not been polished away. It may take longer to cook (usually 50 minutes to an hour), but the improved taste, not to mention the food value, will be well worth a little preplanning. For a different taste, use vegetable or beef stock in place of the water called for in the package instructions. Also, brown rice is much easier to cook (even though it takes longer). Unlike white rice, which can be tricky, brown rice won't get sticky or mushy.

Your Water Supply

Have your water supply tested. If it is found to be overloaded with chemicals and toxins, switch to distilled water. In most cases, it tastes far superior to tap water, especially since it does not have the strong chlorine taste and odor. If you use spring water, which is normally rich in minerals, have this tested as well. Using distilled water may necessitate the addition of mineral supplements to your diet.

Pasta Products

Pasta products may be another area where change can be facilitated. Since most pastas used in American homes are made from refined flour, a change to whole wheat, Jerusalem artichoke and semolina flour-based pastas will net you an increased vitamin source. Although these pastas do not look quite as appetizing at first to a conditioned taste and eye appeal, they really are most delicious and do not overcook as readily as white flour pastas.

Sweet Substitutes

While you are cutting back on refined sugar, you might be wondering what will take its place if you are one of those people who is a victim of a "sweet tooth." Although saccharrin and similar artificial sweeteners have been used for many years by diabetics, recent government research may prove these substances to be harmful if ingested in large quantities over a long period of time. An alternative to both refined sugar and artificial sweeteners might be blackstrap molasses (high in iron and minerals), honey, date or barley malt sweetener. The latter has a pleasant texture and taste, and does not leave the familiar bitter after-taste common in most artificial sweeteners. Don't worry about not getting enough sugar in your diet. It has been estimated that the "hidden sugar" found in most canned products and cereals more than makes up for any you might be missing. If you use molasses, be careful to brush your teeth soon afterwards to prevent tooth decay.

Legumes

For added protein sources, begin building a supply of legumes (peas, beans, and lentils). The protein found in legumes is different from red meat protein, but for many, it is much easier to metabolize and is easier on the system than protein from flesh. Recipes for using legumes in many delicious soups can be found in the recipe section.

Cookware and Utensils

Your cookware and cooking utensils are something you might like to think about. Teflon™ and aluminum have been found to be harmful in the long run. The best cookware health-wise is glass, ceramic, stainless steel, Corning Ware™, clay, copper, and terracotta. There's no need to rush out and buy all new pots and pans immediately, but when the time comes to replace your current set, you might shop around for one of the above-mentioned types. Wooden utensils seem to be the best for a number of reasons, but mainly because they are a natural product and do not get hot. A stainless steel vegetable steamer is another good kitchen "gadget" that you will probably use more and more once you get used to it. A pottery steamer to which no water is added is another good investment, but these are sometimes quite expensive. When you do steam vegetables, remember to save the remaining stock for use in other recipes.

Summary of the Total Glow Program

One More Look at Meditation

In order that you may have one more opportunity to practice meditation, the basic instructions are presented again. Remember that the technique of meditation/relaxation becomes easier and more useful with practice. Your own individual variations will probably enhance your experiences with it, so I encourage you to try different focuses, positions, areas, and locations. On a recent vacation to the seashore, an associate reported that her meditation sessions were exceptionally good; in fact they were much better than they were at home.

So don't be reluctant to experiment with new variations of your meditation routine. It is important to remember that the benefits are cumulative and that the more you meditate regularly on a daily basis, the more relaxed and confident you will be overall. Vacations are an excellent time to meditate, even though you may think that you are not as stressful at these times. To some extent, everyone experiences scurrying thoughts and worries that can be dealt with more effectively through meditation.

One more variation that I might mention involves background sounds or music. Several companies are now marketing devices or recordings that amplify certain sounds such as waves breaking quietly on the seashore or "white" sound, which has been found to be soothing to some people. I have even come across recordings of the sounds a fetus would hear while in the mother's womb, which includes a faint heartbeat. These recordings, if they are pleasant and soothing to you, may aid you in releasing your mind to meditation and prevent you from being distracted by other noises.

The only drawback I can see to these recordings would be that you may become dependent upon them and unable to meditate without them. Even so, you might find them interesting and use them intermittently or on particular occasions.

Here, then, are the basic meditation steps:

1. Find a quiet place to sit where there will be few interruptions.
2. Loosen tight clothing, remove your shoes if you wish, or simply wear a comfortable robe or caftan.
3. Sit in a comfortable, relaxed position, but try not to slouch or place stress on any part of your body. Your arms should be

relaxed and in your lap, on your legs, or on the arms of your chair.
4. Let your eyes close. Take two or three deep breaths and exhale slowly. Beginning with your toes, gradually relax each muscle of your body. Let your head bend forward gently, if that is comfortable. To enhance relaxation of muscle groups, many of my clients benefit from tensing the muscles, then letting them go completely limp. (Many people also benefit from using a special deep breathing technique all day long. Inhale deeply and hold it for the count of two seconds, saying to yourself, "One thousand one, one thousand two..." This counting results in slower, more consistent breathing. Exhale out as deeply as you can for a count of six. Repeat this exercise three times. Use it whenever you feel tense, anxious, light-headed, or angry. The results are quick and rewarding.)

Relax your toes, your feet, ankles, calves, knees, thighs, buttocks, stomach, the small of your back, your chest, shoulders, arms, hands, fingers, neck, facial muscles, and scalp.
5. Begin to hear your focus and let it repeat itself in your mind.

Working Exercise Into Your Life

In summary of the exercise portion of the Total Glow program, the most important thing to remember would be to *think exercise* as much as possible. Some suggestions for turning a sedentary lifestyle into an active one have been provided in this book, but with a little imagination you can come up with many more. Try to remember that when you are inactive you tend to feel lazier and have less energy, simply because your muscles are slowly deteriorating. It doesn't seem to make sense in the beginning, but this is the best suggestion I can make; if you are feeling "down" or exhausted, get up and get moving. Stand up and do a few deep knee bends, toe touches, or jog in place for a minute or two. Take a few deep breaths.

When we start dragging it is usually because our minds are tired and muddled, not our bodies. As mentioned previously, the human body is designed to be more like a marathon runner than a desk worker. Your body is capable of a great deal more activity than you might think. When you do not allow it to function properly by not getting enough exercise, you are really cheating yourself. Weak muscles and a flabby body do nothing for your self-esteem. Once you start moving and being active again, you will notice an increase in mental clarity. This is why it is so beneficial to move around, even when we seem to be tired. Joggers report that even when they feel bushed and exhausted, running helps restore energy and alertness so that the fatigue disappears.

If you work in an office, one other thing you might consider would be discussing your Total Glow program with your employer, asking if you might have a few more minutes for lunch so that you can walk or jog during the day. When employers and supervisors realize that improved health of their employees will net *them* rewards through improved efficiency and reduction of sick leave, most are very much in favor of allowing extra time. Some large companies have even instituted programs where employees are actively encouraged to exercise, meditate, and improve their diets. Perhaps your employer might be in favor of such a program, too.

Helping Your Family to be Happier and Healthier

With your family, I must remind you to approach the whole subject of self-improvement slowly with caution. Children are usually quite receptive to new things, if you can make them appear to be a game or something that is fun. Young children will probably not understand health philosophies, but they can readily understand your loving concern for their welfare. Sometimes older children and spouses can be very reluctant to change their established ways of doing things. Most people feel comfortable with foods that they grew up with. One of the most common complaints regarding healthful foods is: "But I've been eating white bread all my life and it hasn't hurt me." Don't try to argue with your family when they present you with this rationale. Simply tell them that they might enjoy nutritional foods and that they are known to be better for them, so what is the harm in trying? If you can use your creativity and imagination in preparing meals and snacks that are healthful, chances are good that no one will have any long-term objections, especially after seeing how delicious the nutritional foods can be.

I would advise against trying to trick your family into consuming healthful foods. A great many mistakes have been made through serving foods and then saying triumphantly, "That was health food and you didn't even know the difference, did you?" Other people have undone all their efforts by slipping powdered supplements into their family's food, or sneakily trying to get them to eat things they don't like. If you are discovered in a deceptive act like this, you risk even greater rebellion, since your family will feel controlled and deceived. Don't do it.

If you can't get their cooperation, just drop the subject. Go ahead and eat the things that you want to eat while they eat their favorite things. As gradually as possible, you can stop buying the junk foods and start replacing them with things your family does enjoy but that are better for them. I firmly believe that as time goes by we will see a reduction in the additives and preservatives contained in foods.

I also believe that as further research is performed in the area of nutrition we will see that the arguments against health foods will diminish. In my mind there is no doubt that healthy eating can greatly improve your health, your emotional state, your outlook on life, your amount of energy, and, of course, your self-esteem. I sincerely hope that by this time you are of the same persuasion, and can join me in the quest for total health and total glow.

The following are worksheets whereby you can discover those areas where improvement is needed, and to help you design your own Total Glow program specifically for your needs.

Day 4 Implementing The Plan 177

Weight/Body Shape/Muscle Tone

1. I want to lose/gain _____ pounds.
2. The areas of my body that need special attention are: (check as many as apply)

_____ neck   _____ hips
_____ upper arms   _____ backs of thighs
_____ chest (rib area/midriff) _____ sides of thighs
_____ stomach   _____ knees
_____ waistline   _____ calves
_____ buttocks   _____ ankles
                      _____ other _____

Below are drawings of male and female figures. Circle those areas where you feel you need to pay the most attention.

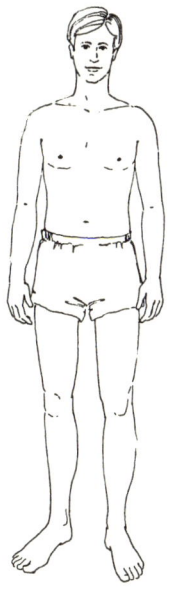
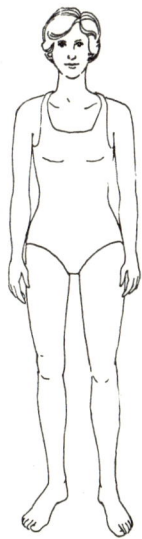

3. I would like to improve my muscle tone in the following areas: (check as many as apply)

   _____ neck   _____ buttocks
   _____ upper arms   _____ hips
   _____ shoulders   _____ thighs
   _____ midriff   _____ calves
   _____ waistline   _____ ankles
   _____ stomach   _____ back
                          _____ other _____

4. Read over the exercises illustrated earlier and choose those that would be most beneficial for the areas circled on your drawing:
   1.
   2.
   3.
   4.
   5.
   6.
   7.
   8.
   9.
   10.

5. Based on the previously listed exercises, the following is an exercise plan I have devised for myself which will benefit my problem areas (Note: If you are your perfect weight, all the exercises will be beneficial in promoting overall muscle tone, enhanced circulatory, digestive, and respiratory functions. They are also good warm-up exercises prior to aerobics).

6. I plan to perform the above exercises _____ times per day/week.
7. In addition to these exercises, I plan to adopt the following "desk" or at-home exercises described previously, and perform them whenever I think of them:

8. In order to get more activity into my life, I would like to do the following things more often (check all that apply):
   _____ Take a walk during the day at least _____ times per week.
   _____ Take a walk in the evening at least _____ times per week.
   _____ Walk up a flight of stairs at a brisk pace at least _____ times per week.
   _____ Enroll in an exercise class that meets _____ times per week.
   _____ Pick out my favorite records and do some general exercising at least _____ times per week.
   _____ Learn and practice the following sport or aerobic exercise regularly:
   _____ tennis   _____ golf (no cart or caddie)
   _____ swimming   _____ handball/squash
   _____ dancing   _____ horseback riding
   _____ bicycling   _____ jogging
   _____ other _____
   _____ I can do the following errands/chores for myself instead of letting my secretary/family get all the exercise:
   _____ getting my own food and drinks (including coffee breaks)
   _____ dropping off/picking up laundry/mail/tickets, etc.
   _____ vacuuming the carpets
   _____ washing/waxing the car
   _____ mowing the lawn
   _____ raking leaves/grounds work
   _____ providing door-to-door chauffer service
   _____ shoveling snow
   _____ general housework/maintenance, etc.

9. I would like to make the following adjustments to my working space so that I have to get up out of my chair more often throughout the day:

10. The following are some other ideas that I may be able to adopt to get more physical activity into my life:

Nutrition/Diet

1. Right now, my diet consists mainly of: (check one)
   _____ junk food
   _____ processed heat-and-serve foods
   _____ reasonably balanced diet with lots of meats, fish, poultry, vegetables, fruits, dairy products, and grains
   _____ a reducing diet   Type: _____
   _____ a special diet   Type: _____
   _____ a mixture of all or most of the above
2. Some of the ways in which I can upgrade my diet are:

3. My number one "weakness" when it comes to food is:

4. One of the ways I might get around over-indulging in this weakness would be:

5. Five of the easiest changes I can personally make to improve my nutrition are:
   1.
   2.
   3.
   4.
   5.

6. If I don't live alone, five of the easiest changes to make with my family to improve nutrition are:
   1.
   2.
   3.
   4.
   5.

Day 4 Implementing The Plan

7. If I want to improve my total health, five things that I can learn to avoid are:
   1.
   2.
   3.
   4.
   5.

8. The recipes I would most like to try in this book are:

9. Similar foods that I might be able to prepare in this manner would be:

10. I have looked up the name, address, and phone number of a local health food store. I plan to visit it on _____ (day) _____ (month) _____ (time)

Meditation/Relaxation

1. When I first heard of meditation, I thought

2. Now that I've learned more about it, I think

3. The results of my first meditation experience were:

4. During my first session of meditating, I was in the following:
   _____room
   _____chair
   _____clothes
   _____mood

5. During my first session of meditating, I was (check those that apply):
   _____ bothered by noise/outside interruptions
   _____ uncomfortable
   _____ amused/skeptical

____ unable to meditate
____ unable to relax
____ surprised by how I felt afterwards
____ eager to meditate again

6. I think my meditation experience might be enhanced by:
____ moving to another room
____ sitting in a more comfortable position
____ wearing ear plugs to block out noise
____ changing my focus
____ taking longer to relax before hearing my focus
____ other _____

7. If you noticed that certain thoughts seemed to be crowding your focus out of your mind and taking over, use this space to jot these thoughts down:

8. While participating in the Total Glow program, I intend to practice meditation ____ times per day/week at the following times ____ a.m. and/or ____ p.m.

9. I would like to meditate before/after exercising.

10. The way I felt after my first successful meditating experience could best be described as:

11. Psychologically, some of the ways I can improve my outlook on life are:

These self-testing questions were included to give you a deeper understanding of your current attitudes, goals, and experiences. You might find it particularly interesting to make extra copies of the questions before you fill them in so that you can complete the questionnaire every so often as you progress through your program. One reason why people have been such avid diary-keepers is that it is so interesting to read back over their writings later on. Try and see what you can learn about yourself by keeping a journal.

The Total Glow Health Barometer

The following barometer is a means of helping you become more in touch with your own health in an objective way. You have already read questions to help you think about yourself more. Now I would like to offer something a little more concrete and an objective way to rate your own physical and emotional health.

Fill in this chart several times a day. I would suggest that you begin in the morning, then jot down your answers again in mid-morning, mid-afternoon, evening, and mid-evening. By recording your feelings at these different times of day, you will become more aware of how you are feeling throughout your regular day. You can also correlate feelings in sequences of prior to and after eating, what you have eaten, and how much.

Use the barometer once a week for a few weeks, then wait a month and go back and fill it in again. Chances are that you will see an increase in good feelings about yourself the longer you practice the Total Glow program.

Some positive changes may not occur immediately, as your body needs time to adjust. If you are cutting things out of your diet immediately (like sugar), you might not feel too good about it. Remember that addictions are hard to kick. But the Total Glow you will achieve after freeing yourself from destructive habits will more than make up for any initial discomfort.

Give yourself the number that most closely describes you in the column at right. Scoring is as follows:
1—Always applies to me.
2—Usually applies to me.
3—Sometimes applies to me.
4—Almost never applies to me.
5—Never applies to me.
The lower your score, the better

1. I accept responsibility and know my own limitations. _____
2. I feel a wonderful zest for living _____
3. I enjoy my work _____
4. I am able to share problems with close friends _____
5. I am comfortable in groups of people _____
6. I am enthusiastic _____
7. I am self-confident _____
8. I am serene _____

9. I can accept and believe compliments from people   _____
10. I appreciate and enjoy nature   _____
11. I am happy   _____
12. I am tolerant of other's mistakes   _____
13. I feel good about my eating habits   _____
14. I carry through on important assignments   _____
15. I am happy with my sex life   _____
16. I have a general, all-around good feeling   _____
17. I like my exercise habits   _____
18. I am flexible when necessary   _____
19. I am able to enjoy myself either alone or with others   _____
20. I am pleased with my life style   _____
21. I enjoy physical contact with both sexes (handshakes, hugs, embraces)   _____
22. I am able to ask for what I want   _____
23. I am aware of my wants and needs   _____
24. I look forward to each day   _____
25. I am able to relax when I need or want to   _____
26. I am able to understand my mistakes and learn from them   _____
27. I can ask questions when necessary   _____
28. I like myself   _____
29. I am able to accept the ups and downs in my life   _____
30. I am a good listener   _____
31. I can accept appropriate criticism without becoming angry or defensive   _____

                                TOTAL   _____

As you will be able to see, you have certain areas where you have a particularly high score. This means that these are the areas where you will need to be more receptive to change. See if you can discover a pattern.

The lower your overall score, the more progress you are making. Enjoy this learning experience and try to recognize where these "trouble spots" might be.

Following is a second group of questions. On these, the same scoring applies, but the higher the score, the better.

1. I have difficulty concentrating _____
2. I do not like to accept responsibility _____
3. I procrastinate _____
4. My feelings are easily hurt _____
5. I complain alot _____
6. I act picky or nag _____
7. I feel disgusted with myself _____
8. I feel light-headed often _____
9. I am dizzy sometimes _____
10. I am confused alot _____
11. I act in a curt manner with people _____
12. I over-react to small things _____
13. I am depressed more than I want to be _____
14. I feel anxious _____
15. I blame others frequently _____
16. I am afraid or feel threatened _____
17. I am worried _____
18. I am restless and fidgety _____
19. I am discouraged _____
20. I use alcohol or drugs to excess _____
21. I am lonely _____
22. I give in to others too soon _____
23. I feel guilty _____
24. I have certain phobias (irrational fears) _____
25. I have difficulty saying "no" when I want to _____
26. I am explosive _____
27. I feel nervous _____
28. I have one of the following symptoms: headaches, skin disorders, nervous disorders, diarrhea, rapid heart beat, constipation _____
29. I tend to hold grudges _____
30. I harbor anger at myself for past mistakes _____
                                                  TOTAL _____

Introduction to the Recipes

The following recipes have been developed through years of testing and experimenting in my own kitchen. As mentioned previously, men have been found to be quite adept in the kitchen, and they are encouraged to give it a try. Any good cookbook (such as *The Joy of Cooking*) will provide you with many of the rudiments of working in the kitchen if you are not familiar with them, along with many definitions of the processes involved.

Starting with simple breakfast dishes, I will take you through luncheon suggestions, main dishes, salads, soups, dips and condiments, breads, desserts, and end with a menu plan and party suggestions. I urge you to try as many of these delicious and easy recipes as appeal to you.

The recipes with asterisks are ones that are particularly good if you are desirous of losing weight. These are either low in calories or carbohydrates and starches.

Remember the basic guidelines for using organically grown food, are to use fresh ingredients, and additive-free products as much as possible.

Breakfast
*Scrambled Eggs** *(low calorie)*
Servings: 4
Ingredients:

> 1 teaspoon melted butter
> ¼ cup chopped onion (more, if desired)
> 2 tablespoons chopped green pepper
> 2 cloves garlic, minced
> 8 eggs
> ½ cup milk
> ¼ teaspoon cayenne pepper ⎤
> ¼ teaspoon sea salt   ⎬ seasonings
> 1 tablespoon tamari   ⎦

Preparation:

Beat together eggs and milk. Melt butter in a large skillet. Saute onion, green peppers, and garlic until onions are clear, but not brown.**

Add egg mixture and seasonings.*** Stir until thickened and set to desired consistency.

Variations:

**Sliced fresh mushrooms may be added at this time to sauted onions. You might wish to experiment with other fresh vegetables.

***If desired, add ½ cup of your favorite shredded cheese at this point.

Healthy Egg Muffin
Servings: 1
Ingredients:

> ½ English Muffin (without preservatives) or ½ 7-grain muffin
> 1 poached egg (3 minute)
> 2 tablespoons shredded cheese

Preparation:

Toast muffin. Boil water in a small saucepan, then reduce to simmer. Crack egg in saucer and pour into pan of hot water, poach for 3 minutes. Remove egg with slotted server and let water drain. Place on toasted muffin half, add shredded cheese, and place under broiler for 30 seconds, or until cheese melts.

Basic Omelet(low calorie)*

Servings: 1
Ingredients:

>2 eggs
>¼ teaspoon herbs (dill, oregano, tarragon, chives, thyme, or your favorite)
>dash cayenne pepper
>butter for pan

Preparation:

Beat eggs until fluffy and add herbs and cayenne pepper. Melt about ½ teaspoon butter in the bottom of a pre-heated omelet pan. Swirl, making sure the bottom is covered with melted butter. Pour egg mixture into pan, allowing the mixture to cover bottom. Let set for one minute. As the omelet cooks, pull the edges back with a fork so that the uncooked part slides under. Cook until bottom is golden. Add fillings (see below) if desired, fold omelet in half, and slide onto a warm plate.

Fillings: (if desired)

Cheese—sprinkle 4 tablespoons of your favorite cheese on the inside fold of the omelet. Sprinkle 2 tablespoons of cheese on the top. Place in a pre-heated oven for a few minutes until cheese melts.
Mushroom—Saute 6 sliced mushrooms and ½ a medium onion in 3 tablespoons butter. Insert mixture into the inside fold of the omelet. Sprinkle 2 tablespoons of cheese on the top and place in a pre-heated oven until cheese melts.
Green Peppers and Onions—Saute one small green pepper and ½ a medium onion in 3 tablespoons butter. Insert into the inside fold of the omelet. In season, add 1 small chopped tomato, ½ teaspoon basil, and ¼ teaspoon oregano to green peppers and onions, cooking for a few minutes longer.

Whole Wheat Pancakes

Servings: 4–5 6" pancakes

Ingredients:

    1¼ cups freshly ground whole wheat flour
    3 tablespoons butter, melted and cooled
    2 eggs
    1½ teaspoons baking powder
    1 cup milk, buttermilk, sour milk, or orange juice

Preparation:

    Beat eggs until light and fluffy, add milk and butter. Mix in flour and baking powder. Bake on a lightly buttered griddle, using medium heat. The pancake is ready to be turned when bubbles appear. Flip over and bake on the other side.

    Serve with low-calorie maple syrup, honey, or your favorite fruit preserves.

Homemade Sausage* (low calorie)

Servings: 12 patties

Ingredients:

    1 pound ground lamb
    1 teaspoon dried sage, ground
    1 teaspoon seasoning salt (recipe included)
    ¼ teaspoon papaya pepper
    ½ teaspoon dried thyme, ground
    ½ teaspoon dried marjoram, ground
    ¼ teaspoon dried cayenne pepper, ground
    2 cloves garlic, minced**

Preparation:

    Place all ingredients in a large mixing bowl. Squeeze and mix thoroughly with your hands until herbs are well-blended. Shape into patties in desired size and thickness.

    Broil about five inches from flame or element for about five minutes on each side until done to your liking.

These patties can be frozen before cooking for future use. If frozen, increase cooking time accordingly.

**When "cloves" of garlic are mentioned, we refer to the *separate sections* (like an orange) of the whole bulb of garlic as you buy it in the store.

Homemade Cereal

Ingredients:

Select one pound of any of the following ingredients, or one pound of a combination of any four.

wheat berries	*mung beans*
buckwheat	*rye*
oat groats	*flax seeds*
barley	*alfalfa*
brown rice	*corn*
pop corn	*chia seeds*
millet	*almonds*

Add one pound sesame seeds.

Preparation:

In a large container, mix together your choice of at least four of the above ingredients. Store in refrigerator or freeze in small containers. Twenty-four hours before eating, remove from storage and place 3 or 4 tablespoons per serving of the mixture in a blender or seed mill.

Grind, cover with milk and refrigerate. Allow to soak for 24 hours. Use within three days or less.

Serve with any fresh fruits, nuts, honey, or fruit concentrate.

High Energy Cereal

Servings: 3

Ingredients: *all whole grains*

8 tablespoons whole wheat berries
6 tablespoons barley
4 tablespoons oats

4 tablespoons millet
3 tablespoons rye
½ cup figs, prunes, raisins, currants, dates, or apples (optional)

Preparation:

Place the whole grains in a large bowl and mix thoroughly. Lightly crack grains in a seed mill or flour grinder (do not pulverize or make into flour).

Place ground mixture into a pot with a tight-fitting lid. Add hot water to cover, and mix until mixture is elastic and loose. Add dried fruit, if desired.

Pour mixture into a baking dish and place in 180° oven. Bake for 30 minutes to two hours, depending on your preference.

Remove from oven and add 2 tablespoons honey. Serve with milk.

Nutrition Drink
Servings: 1

Ingredients:

½ cup apple juice
½ cup frozen raspberry yogurt
2 fresh eggs
½ cup crushed ice

Preparation:

Place all ingredients in a blender and blend at high speed for about 1 minute. Garnish with sprinkles of granola or crushed nuts. Serve for breakfast, snack, or with dinner.

Fruit Nutrition Drink
Servings: 2

Ingredients:

1 apple, cored
1 orange, peeled
1 banana, peeled
2 eggs

Introduction to the Recipes 193

Preparation:

Slice fruit, combine with eggs in blender or food processor, and blend until smooth in consistency. If too thick, add a few tablespoons of yogurt, milk, or fruit juice.

Yogurt Shakes

Servings: 1

Ingredients:

Juices:	Yogurts:
orange	*strawberry*
pineapple	*raspberry*
apricot	*banana*
peach	*carob*
coconut	*vanilla*
grape	*almond crunch*
black cherry	*lime*
apple	
banana	

Preparation:

Select one juice and one yogurt from the two columns above. Use ¼ cup juice to ½ cup yogurt. Add ½ cup chopped ice to blender, juice and yogurt, and blend at high speed until foamy.

Pour into tall glass and garnish with granola, ground nuts, or coconut.

For breakfast, add one or two eggs per person.

Sandwich/Luncheon

Tuna Salad Sandwich

Servings: 4

Ingredients:

1 6½ oz. can of water packed tuna, drained
2 scallions, chopped finely
½ cup celery, chopped finely
1 teaspoon dried dill

>   3 tablespoons fresh parsley, chopped finely
>   6 tablespoons mayonnaise, thinned with few drops lemon juice

Preparation:

Drain tuna and flake with a fork. Add the remaining ingredients and toss lightly to coat. Spread on whole grain bread, with romaine lettuce or fresh spinach.

Variations:

Add 1 grated carrot, 1 small grated zucchini, or 1 grated cucumber, and serve as a salad or sandwich filling with some fresh sprouts.

Spread some of the tuna mixture on ½ an English muffin, top with slice of cheese, and place under broiler until cheese is melted and bubbly.

Homemade Peanut Butter and Jelly Sandwich

Servings: 1

Ingredients:

>   4 tablespoons homemade peanut butter (see recipe below)
>   2 tablespoons fruit jelly (made from organically grown fruit)
>   2 slices whole wheat bread

Preparation:

Spread peanut butter on bread, top with jelly and remaining slice of bread.

Homemade Peanut Butter

Servings: 1½ cups

Ingredients:

>   2 cups raw, shelled peanuts
>   ½ cup oil (sesame, safflower, etc.)

Preparation:

Spread the peanuts in a shallow pan and roast in a 350° oven for about 30 minutes, or until brown. Allow to cool and remove skins. They will usually come off easily by rubbing the peanuts between your hands.

Place peanuts in an electric blender and blend for two minutes. Gradually add oil, blending thoroughly. Keep peanut butter stored in a glass jar in the refrigerator.

Vegetarian Carrot Sandwich

Servings: 4 to 6

Ingredients:

> *1 grated carrot*
> *½ cup chopped walnuts*
> *½ cup raisins*
> *½ cup celery, chopped finely*
> *½ cup mayonnaise, thinned with a few drops of lemon juice*
> *4 tablespoons yogurt*
> *Dried dill to taste*

Preparation:

Place first 4 ingredients in bowl and mix. Add mayonnaise and yogurt, tossing lightly to coat. Gradually add dill to taste.

Spread on whole wheat bread. Serve with raw green pepper strips.

*Peanut and Raisin Snack** *(low calorie)*

Ingredients:

> *2 lbs. raw, shelled, unsalted peanuts*
> *1 lb. sultana raisins*

Preparation:

Roast peanuts in a 350° oven until nicely browned (about 30 minutes). Mix with raisins and store in a glass jar in the refrigerator.

Variations:

Add sunflower seeds, sesame seeds, shredded coconut, dates, or other dried fruit. Substitute other raw nuts for peanuts.

*McGuckin Special** (low calorie)
Servings: 4

Ingredients:

> fresh, organically-grown apples
> natural peanut butter (homemade)

Preparation:

Cut fresh apples into quarters or eighths so that you have bite-size wedges. Remove and discard core sections.

Dab a small amount of peanut butter on each wedge and you have a great snack or simple dessert that is especially enjoyed by youngsters.

Dips and Condiments

*Elaine's Dill Dip** (low calorie)

Ingredients:

> ½ cup yogurt
> 1 cup low-fat cottage cheese
> ½ cup mayonnaise
> 1 heaping teaspoon dill weed
> 3 tablespoons fresh mint, minced (optional)
> 2 tablespoons parsley
> 1 teaspoon Beau Monde seasoning

Preparation:

Place all ingredients in a blender and blend at high speed until thoroughly mixed. Serve chilled with raw vegetables.

Avocado Dip

Ingredients:

    2 ripe avocadoes, peeled and seeded
    3 tablespoons lemon juice
    ½ teaspoon kelp
    ½ teaspoon chili powder
    2 tablespoons ketchup
    ¼ cup mayonnaise–or–¼ cup low-fat cottage cheese
    1 onion, grated

Preparation:

Combine all ingredients in a blender. Blend at low speed until smooth. To store in refrigerator, cover with a thin layer of mayonnaise to prevent darkening, in a tightly sealed container.

Anchovy Dip

Ingredients:

    1 cup low-fat cottage cheese
    ¼ cup raw cream or buttermilk
    1 can anchovies with oil
    2 scallions, including greens, chopped finely

Preparations:

Place all ingredients in a blender. Blend at low speed until smooth. Serve chilled.

Bleu Cheese Salad Dressing or Dip

Ingredients:

    1 8oz. carton plain yogurt
    ½ cup crumbled Bleu cheese
    2 tablespoons skim milk or buttermilk
    salad dressing mix (organic, without preservatives)

Preparation:

Place all ingredients in a blender and blend at low speed until smooth and mixed thoroughly. Serve as a salad dressing or dip.

Variations:

For Italian dressing, follow above directions and add one packet organic Italian dressing mix. Blend to desired consistency.

Onion Dip

Ingredients:

> ½ cup plain yogurt
> ½ cup cottage cheese
> 3 tablespoons organic onion seasoning

Preparation:

Blend all ingredients at low speed in blender. Store in refrigerator for at least ½ hour before serving.

Tarter Sauce

Ingredients:

> ½ cup mayonnaise
> 1 teaspoon capers
> ½ cup grated onion
> ½ cup dill weed

Preparation:

Combine all ingredients in a blender. Blend at low speed until smooth. Chill before serving.

Barbeque Sauce

Ingredients:

    1 *8oz. bottle ketchup (sweetened with honey, preservative-free)*
    ½ *cup vinegar*
    1 *medium onion, sliced*
    1 *lemon, thinly sliced*
    1 *clove garlic, mashed*
    2 *teaspoons mustard*
    1½ *teaspoons Worcestershire sauce*

Preparation:

Put all ingredients in a saucepan and bring to a boil. Simmer 15 to 20 minutes, stirring ocassionally. Store in refrigerator.

Blender Mayonnaise

Ingredients:

    2 egg yolks–or–1 whole egg
    1 tablespoon lemon juice
    1 tablespoon cider vinegar
    ¼ teaspoon salt (optional)
    ½ teaspoon dry mustard
    1⅓ cups oil

Preparation:

Combine all ingredients except oil. Pour into blender and blend for about 1 minute.

Slowly but continuously add oil and blend until all oil is integrated into mixture. Scrape the sides of the blender often.

Pour mayonnaise into glass container and store tightly covered in refrigerator.

Homemade Ketchup

Ingredients:

> 3 6oz. cans tomato paste (unsalted)
> 1 #2½ can tomato puree
> ½ cup vinegar
> 2 tablespoons molasses
> 2 tablespoons honey
> 1 teaspoon allspice
> ½ teaspoon cloves
> 2 tablespoons onions, grated
> 4 cloves garlic, crushed
> 1 to 1½ teaspoons seasoning salt (optional)
> few dashes Worchestershire sauce or Tobasco sauce

Preparation:

Blend all ingredients thoroughly and store tightly sealed in refrigerator until ready to use.

Herbal Seasoning Salt

Ingredients:

> ⅛ cup sea salt
> ⅛ cup kelp
> 1 tablespoon dried parsley
> 1½ teaspoons dried celery
> ½ teaspoon onion powder
> 1 teaspoon paprika
> ⅛ teaspoon cayenne
> ½ teaspoon dried thyme
> ½ teaspoon marjoram
> 1 teaspoon ground, toasted sesame seeds

Preparation:

Place all ingredients in a blender. Touch blend button for a few seconds, until all ingredients are well-mixed. Store in herb shaker, away from heat.

Use this as a salt-substitute or to help get away from table salt.

Soups

Easy Lentil Soup

Servings: 6

Ingredients:

> 2 cups lentils (organic, preservative-free)
> 6 cups vegetable or chicken stock–or–6 tablespoons powdered base with 6 to 7 cups water
> 2 one-pound cans tomatoes (unsalted) with juice
> 1 medium onion, finely chopped
> 2 to 3 teaspoons garlic, minced
> sea salt to taste (optional)
> ½ teaspoon ground cumin
> 1 teaspoon parsley
> 1 teaspoon parakelp
> cayenne pepper to taste

Preparation:

Combine stock, onions, garlic. Cook over medium heat in a slow cooker for 1 hour. Add lentils, tomatoes, juice, cumin, sea salt, and parsley. Cook an additional 2 hours. Add additional cumin and sea salt to taste.

*Gazpacho** (low calorie)

Ingredients:

> 2 cucumbers, peeled, seeded, and coarsley chopped
> 6 tomatoes, peeled, coarsely chopped
> 1 green pepper, seeded and cored, chopped
> 1 large onion, chopped
> 2½ teaspoons garlic, finely chopped
> 2 cups cold water
> ¼ cup red wine vinegar
> 1½ teaspoons sea salt (optional)
> 1 teaspoon cayenne
> 3 tablespoons olive oil
> 2 tablespoons tomato paste (unsalted)
> 1 tablespoon lemon juice

Preparation:

In a large bowl, combine cucumbers, tomatoes, onions, green pepper, and garlic. Mix thoroughly. Stir in water, salt, vinegar, and cayenne. Ladle about one cup at a time into blender, and puree until smooth. Pour puree into a bowl and beat in olive oil and tomato paste with a wire whisk.

Cover the bowl tightly and chill for at least 2 hours. Just before serving, stir well to combine all ingredients thoroughly.

Garnish with chopped onions, chopped cucumbers, chopped green pepper, or bread cubes. Add cubed avocado in season.

Carol and Luanne's Onion Soup

Servings: 6 to 8

Ingredients:

    4 tablespoons butter
    4 tablespoons oil
    3 pounds onions, thinly sliced
    1 teaspoon sea salt (optional)
    3 to 5 tablespoons unbleached flour
    2 quarts beef or vegetable stock
    1 loaf French bread
    2 cloves garlic, sliced
    ½ cup grated Swiss or Parmesan cheese

Preparation:

In a large saucepan, melt butter and oil. Stir in onions and salt. Cook uncovered on low heat, stirring occasionally for 20 to 30 minutes, until onions are golden brown.

In another large saucepan, bring stock to a simmer, then stir into onions. Simmer, partially covered for 40 minutes or longer. Skim off fat. Add salt and cayenne pepper to taste.

Slice the loaf of French bread and spread each slice with oil. Brown in a 325° oven for 10 to 15 minutes, then rub both sides of each slice with garlic.

Place toasted bread slices in individual soup bowls and fill with hot soup. Sprinkle cheese over top and heat in moderate oven for 10 to 15 minutes. Serve at once, piping hot.

Pat's Paradise Soup

Servings: 6 to 8

Ingredients:

    4 to 5 cups Tomato Juice Mix (see page 216) or V-8 Juice
    1 cup plain yogurt
    2 tablespoons lemon juice
    sea salt and cayenne pepper to taste
    ¾ cup diced ham
    2 medium cucumbers, cubed
    1 medium cantalope and/or honeydew melon, scooped into balls
    pinch basil

Preparation:

    Combine the first 5 ingredients in a bowl and chill for at least 4 hours. Add cucumbers and cantalope and return to refrigerator to chill for another 4 hours. Sprinkle with basil just before serving to garnish.

Pea Soup

Ingredients:

    2   cups split peas (organic, preservative free)
    5   cups water
    1   ham bone
    1   to 1½ cups chopped onion
    3   cloves garlic, minced
    1   cup celery, coarsley chopped
    1½ cups carrots, thinly sliced
    2   cups potatoes with skins, diced (optional)
    ⅓   cup green pepper, chopped
    1   tablespoon parsley, chopped
    ½   teaspoon oregano, chopped
    1   teaspoon parakelp
    ½   teaspoon cumin

Preparation:

    Rinse peas in a collander and soak for 2 hours in water. Place them with water and ham bone in a large saucepan and cook over medium heat for about 1 hour, stirring frequently to avoid sticking. Add remaining ingredients and cook for another hour. Serve hot.

If you use a slow cooker, place peas and water and ham bone in pot and cook over medium heat for approximately 2 hours. Add all remaining ingredients except for potatoes and cook another 3 hours. Add potatoes and cook 1 more hour. Serve hot.

Bean Soup

Ingredients:

> 2 to 2½ cups beans (organic, preservative free)
> 5 to 6 cups water
> 1 ham bone
> 1 cup onions, chopped
> 2 cloves garlic, minced
> ¼ cup green pepper, chopped
> 1 cup carrots, chopped
> 1 tablespoon parsley, chopped
> ½ teaspoon oregano
> 1 teaspoon parakelp
> ½ teaspoon cumin
> ½ to 1 teaspoon sea salt (optional)

Preparation:

Rinse beans and place them in large pot, along with water, ham bone, onions, garlic, celery, green pepper, and carrots.

Cook over low heat for about 1½ hours, stirring occasionally. Add seasonings and cook for another 1½ hours.

If using a slow cooker, add all ingredients at once and double cooking time to about 6 hours over medium heat.

Hearty Vegetable Soup

Servings: 8 to 10

Ingredients:

- 2 to 3 pounds pot roast or chuck steak, cut into 1" cubes, fat removed (optional)
- 4 cups water
- 4 to 6 cloves garlic, minced
- 1½ cups onions, coarsley chopped
- 2 cups celery, cut into ½" slices
- 2 one-pound cans tomatoes (unsalted)
- 2 cups carrots, cut into ½" slices
- 2 cups fresh string beans, sliced
- 1 to 2 cups peas
- ½ cup turnips, cut into ½" cubes
- ½ cup rutabaga, cut into ½" cubes
- ½ to 1 cup beets, cubed
- 1 to 2 cups potatoes, cubed
- 3 tablespoons vegetable soup base (powdered)
- 1 tablespoon beef soup base (powdered)
- 1 tablespoon chicken soup base (powdered)
- 1 tablespoon fresh parsley
- 1 tablespoon mixed Italian seasoning
- 1 tablespoon parakelp
- 1 teaspoon sea salt (optional)
- ½ teaspoon cayenne pepper

Preparation:

Place cubed meat in a slow cooker along with water and cook at medium heat for about an hour. Add garlic, onions, celery, and cook for another hour. Add all remaining vegetables, except potatoes, and cook for an additional 4 hours on medium heat. Add herbs, seasonings, and potatoes, and cook another 1 to 2 hours.

Salads

Macaroni and Tuna Salad
Servings: 6 to 8

Ingredients:

    1½ cups wheat and soy macaroni**
    1 cup mayonnaise (or ½ cup mayonnaise and ½ cup yogurt)
    juice of ½ a lemon
    1½ tablespoons fresh snipped dill (or 1 tablespoon dried)
    ½ teaspoon fresh basil (or ¼ teaspoon dried)
    ¼ teaspoon cayenne pepper
    2 tablespoons relish***
    4 scallions, thinly sliced
    ½ cup celery, chopped
    ¼ cup parsley, chopped
    1 13oz. can water-pack tuna, drained
    1 cup lightly steamed peas

Preparation:

    Cook macaroni in boiling water for about 6 to 8 minutes and drain well. Blend together mayonnaise, dill, basil, pepper, and relish. Stir into macaroni. Add the scallions, celery, parsley, tuna, and peas, tossing lightly. Chill and serve.

**Pasta products made from durum semolina, soy, and Jerusalem artichoke flours are best to use and can be found at health food stores.

***Purchase relish from health food stores containing no artificial colors or preservatives, and made with honey.

Double Crunch Peanut Salad
Servings: 4 to 6

Ingredients:

    4 cups shredded cabbage
    ½ cup chopped green onions, including tops
    1 cup chopped celery

1 cup chopped peanuts
½ cup almonds
½ cup homemade mayonnaise (or preservative-free)

Preparation:

Toss the cabbage, celery, and nuts together lightly. Stir in enough mayonnaise to moisten well. Chill before serving.

Potato Salad

Servings: 6 to 8

Ingredients:

2 pounds potatoes, unpeeled
½ cup celery, finely chopped
½ cup green pepper, finely chopped
1 small onion, finely chopped
¼ cup parsley, finely chopped
2 hard-boiled eggs, chopped
1 cup mayonnaise
juice of ½ a lemon
1 teaspoon fresh snipped dill (or ½ teaspoon dried)
1 tablespoon prepared mustard
1 teaspoon parakelp

Preparation:

Cook potatoes in boiling water. When cooked, drain and cool. Peel and dice into one-inch pieces.

Place potatoes in a bowl with celery, green pepper, onion, parsley, and eggs. Mix together with mayonnaise, lemon juice, dill, mustard, and parakelp. Toss with potato mixture. Chill. Salad tastes better when allowed to marinate 24 hours. Garnish with more chopped parsley and serve.

Waldorf Salad Ambrosia
Servings: 4

Ingredients:

>1 large red apple, including skin (if organic)
>¾ cup diced pineapple (fresh, frozen, or water-pack)
>¾ cup diced celery
>⅓ cup chopped almonds, walnuts, or pecans (or combination)
>⅔ cup plain yogurt
>2 tablespoons unsweetened coconut, shredded

Preparation:

Core and dice the apple and combine with pineapple, celery, and nuts. Add yogurt and toss lightly. Garnish with coconut.

Marinated Mushrooms* (low calorie)

Ingredients:

>1 pound fresh mushrooms
>½ cup olive oil
>½ cup red wine vinegar
>2 cloves garlic, crushed
>2 tablespoons horseradish
>½ teaspoon oregano
>½ teaspoon sea salt (optional)
>cayenne pepper to taste

Preparation:

Wash mushrooms in cold water. Drop into boiling water and simmer for 5 minutes. Drain

Mix other ingredients in a glass jar and shake well to blend. Add mushrooms and refrigerate overnight. Shake every now and then while storing to prevent liquid from separating.

When mushrooms are gone, use the leftover liquid as a salad dressing, or as a base for salad dressings.

Pineapple Coleslaw(low calorie)*

Ingredients:

> ½ cup fresh pineapple with juice (or 1 can unsweetend water-pack)
> 2 cups shredded cabbage
> ⅓ cup plain yogurt
> ⅛ teaspoon seasoned kelp
> herbal seasoning to taste

Preparation:

Mix all of the above ingredients and toss lightly to coat. Serve with garnishes.

Sweet and Sour Marinated Cucumbers and Onions(low calorie)*

Ingredients:

> 1 large cucumber, peeled and sliced
> 1 medium onion (or ½ a large Spanish onion, sliced)
> ½ to ⅔ cup natural cider vinegar
> 2 to 3 tablespoons honey, barley malt sweetener, or other sweetener, or 3 packets sugar substitute.
> ½ teaspoon parakelp
> ¼ teaspoon cayenne pepper

Preparation:

Combine all the above ingredients, cover, and allow to marinate at room temperature for ½ an hour, or refrigerate and marinate several hours before serving.

When the vegetables are gone, use this liquid as a salad dressing, or as a base for salad dressings.

This recipe is also adaptable to most vegetables. It may be prepared using the cucumbers or onions separately, or shredded cabbage, green pepper, raw cauliflower, or celery.

Cabbage Salad* (low calorie)

Ingredients:

    1 medium green cabbage, finely shredded
    1 cup carrots, finely shredded
    1 cup onion, finely chopped
    ¼ cup fresh parsley, finely chopped
    1 medium apple, cored and diced

Preparation:

    Toss cabbage, carrots, onion, parsley, and apple in mixing bowl. Add a dressing of mayonnaise and yogurt. Serve on individual plates by heaping a mound of this salad on a bed of romaine lettuce or sprouts.

Mayonnaise and Yogurt Dressing

Ingredients:

    ½ cup mayonnaise
    ½ cup plain yogurt
    ½ teaspoon dried tarragon
    ¼ teaspoon kelp seasoning salt (optional)

Preparation:

    Place all ingredients in a small bowl and mix well. Serve chilled.

Yogurt Vinaigrette

Ingredients:

    ¼ teaspoon herbal salt
    ¼ teaspoon kelp seasoning
    1 teaspoon dried mustard
    1 tablespoon fresh lemon juice
    5 tablespoons safflower oil
    5 tablespoons plain yogurt
    2 cloves garlic, minced.

Preparation:

Combine all the ingredients in a screw-top jar, close tightly, and shake mixture until it emulsifies. Store in refrigerator until ready to use.

Raw Mushroom and Herb Salad (low calorie)

Servings: 4 to 6

Ingredients:

>1 pound fresh mushrooms, sliced thickly and stems removed
>1 tablespoon fresh lemon juice
>2 tablespoons scallions, finely chopped
>1 tablespoon fresh tarragon
>1 tablespoon fresh dill
>2 tablespoons fresh parsley, finely chopped
>½ cup yogurt vinaigrette (recipe above)
>few sprigs watercress

Preparation:

Wash the mushrooms in a bowl of cold water with the lemon juice. Combine the sliced mushrooms with the chopped herbs and parsley in a bowl with the yogurt vinaigrette. Marinate in the refrigerator for at least 30 minutes. Serve in a bowl garnished with watercress sprigs.

*Cucumber and Onion Salad**

Servings: 4

Ingredients:

>2 large cucumbers, sliced thinly
>1 medium Bermuda onion, sliced thinly
>cider vinegar
>1 teaspoon basil
>1 teaspoon dill
>1 teaspoon tarragon
>1 teaspoon mint

Preparation:

Place cucumbers in bowl, alternating layers with the onions. Cover with cider vinegar and snip fresh herbs over the mixture. If using dried herbs, mix with the vinegar. Allow to marinate for several hours.

To serve, drain and place mixture on a bed of lettuce, add herbed salt to taste and garnish with a dollop of plain yogurt.

Vegetables

*Stewed Eggplant** (low calorie)

Ingredients:

> 1 large eggplant, peeled and cubed
> 4 large fresh tomatoes, peeled (or 1 one-pound can unsalted tomatoes)
> 1 large onion, coarsely chopped
> 1 green pepper, coarsely chopped
> 2 stalks celery, coarsely chopped
> 2 cloves garlic, crushed
> ½ teaspoon dried basil (or 1 tablespoon fresh basil)
> ½ teaspoon oregano (or 1 tablespoon fresh oregano)
> herbal salt and kelp seasoning to taste

Preparation:

Put all ingredients into a large pot, cover, and cook over medium heat for about 30 minutes.

This recipe can also be adapted to your charcoal grill. Wrap all ingredients in foil and cook for about 45 minutes over flames.

*Yellow Crook Necked Squash** (low calorie)

Ingredients:

> 2 pounds yellow squash, cubed
> 2 medium onions, chopped
> cayenne pepper to taste
> kelp seasoning to taste
> 1 clove garlic

Preparation:

Cut squash into ½" cubes. If skin appears to be tough, peel. Chop onion, slice garlic in half, and add with squash to large skillet. Sprinkle cayenne pepper and kelp seasoning to taste over all.

Cover and cook at medium heat, stirring ocassionally for about 30 minutes, or until tender but still slightly crisp. If squash tends to stick to pan, reduce heat and add a splash of water.

Oven Potatoes

Servings: 4 to 6

Ingredients:

4 medium potatoes with skins
2 medium onions, sliced
butter
organic onion soup (stock) mix
sea salt (optional)

Preparation:

Wash potatoes and slice into ¼" slices. Arrange potatoes on a piece of aluminum foil with a slice of onion between each slice of potato. Dot with butter. Sprinkle with organic onion soup mix, and sea salt.

Wrap in foil and bake in 400° oven for 50 minutes, or on charcoal grill until done.

Roasted Corn

Preparation:

Remove loose husks from fresh ears of corn, making sure the kernels are still well covered with the husks closest to the corn.

Place corn on rack of pre-heated 325° oven, one layer at a time. Bake for 45 minutes. If cooking more than one layer, rearrange so that top and bottom layers are switched mid-way through cooking time.

Husk the corn at the table just before eating, while protecting hands with cloths or towels.

Lightly Steamed Vegetables *(low calorie)*

Wash leafy vegetables retaining water. Chop stems off and place in stainless steel saucepan, then chop leafy section and add on top of stems. Depending on the type of cookware, you may need to add one to three tablespoons of water.

Turn the heat to medium. When the lid will "swirl" (steam has risen to give a cushion of steam under the lid), turn heat as low as possible and steam only long enough to tenderize stems and wilt leafy sections.

If making big batches of vegetables, lift lid and stir vegetables up from the bottom half-way through steaming process.

Chard takes about 4 minutes, squash 10 minutes, green beans about 15 minutes. Steam all vegetable considerably below boiling point, under 180° F. The smaller the pieces the more quickly they cook. Shred beets and other root vegetables to tenderize in less than 5 minutes.

Main Dishes

Broiled Chicken "Italian" *(low calorie)*

Servings: 4

Ingredients:

>6 to 8 pieces of chicken, skinned
>oregano
>crushed garlic
>½ cup Tomato Juice Mix (see page 216)
>¼ to ½ cup grated Parmesean cheese

Preparation:

Place chicken in a pan suitable for broiling, meaty side up. Sprinkle each piece with a pinch of oregano and some garlic. Pour Tomato Juice Mix over chicken and into pan.

Broil for 10 minutes, then turn and broil for about 10 minutes on the other side. In the last 5 minutes of broiling, sprinkle grated cheese on top of chicken and return to broiler until browned.

Lemon Tarragon Chicken*(low calorie)

Servings: 4

Ingredients:

>6 to 8 pieces of chicken, skinned
>tarragon
>cayenne pepper
>½ cup fresh lemon juice

Preparation:

Place chicken in a pan suitable for broiling. Sprinkle each piece with tarragon and cayenne pepper. Add lemon juice to pan.

Broil for 10 minutes, then turn chicken and broil for another 10 minutes, or until browned.

Variations:

Different spices may be added, or you may choose a combination of herbs such as basil, rosemary, thyme, parsley, and paprika. Lemon Tarragon Chicken may also be served chilled as a luncheon or picnic meal.

"Wine Savored" Chicken Breasts*(low calorie)

Servings: 4

Ingredients:

>4 to 6 chicken breasts, skinned
>parsley
>paprika
>2 cloves garlic crushed
>½ cup white wine
>¼ to ½ cup grated Swiss Cheese

Preparation:

Place chicken in pan suitable for broiling. Sprinkle each piece with parsley and paprika. Crush garlic and combine with wine. Pour the wine mixture over chicken and into pan.

Broil for 8 minutes, turn over, and continue broiling for an additional 8 minutes.

In the last 3 minutes of broiling, sprinkle grated cheese on top and return to broiler until browned and bubbly.

Tomato Juice Mix

In a blender, combine preservative-free tomato juice, freshly ground dried papaya seeds or cayenne pepper, sea salt or parakelp to taste, a dash of lime juice, tarragon, and tamari soy sauce. Blend well.

*Chicken Marengo Italiano**

Servings: 4

Ingredients:

>   2 medium chickens, cut into pieces and skinned
>   3 tablespoons olive oil
>   1 large (or 2 medium) onions, chopped
>   4 cloves garlic, minced
>   2 one-pound cans tomatoes, with juice (unsalted)
>   1 tablespoon parsley, minced
>   2 bay leaves
>   1 teaspoon oregano
>   1 teaspoon basil
>   ½ teaspoon thyme
>   ⅔ cup white wine
>   1 teaspoon lemon juice
>   several dashes cayenne pepper
>   ½ to ¾ pound fresh mushrooms

Preparation:

In a 350° oven, bake chicken for 10 minutes on each side.

Place olive oil in a large flameproof skillet, add onion and garlic, and saute until delicately tender, not brown. Add chicken and all of the above ingredients except lemon juice, cayenne pepper, and mushrooms. Heat through.

Return to large baking dish and bake, uncovered, for about 50 minutes, or until chicken is tender.

Add lemon juice, cayenne pepper, and mushrooms. Cook 5 minutes longer.

Variations:

This recipe is adaptable to a slow cooker. After briefly baking chicken, place it and all other ingredients in cooker and cook approximately 8 hours on a low setting.

Roast Lamb With Herbs and Garlic **

Servings: 6 to 8

Ingredients:

1 five-to seven-pound leg of lamb
3 cloves garlic, crushed
1 tablespoon sea salt (optional)
kelp seasoning
1 teaspoon powdered ginger
2 bay leaves, bruised
1 teaspoon thyme
1 teaspoon sage
1 teaspoon marjoram
1 teaspoon rosemary
2 tablespoons tamari soy sauce
2 tablespoons oil

Preparation:

The day before cooking, cut slivers into the flesh of the lamb and insert cloves of garlic. Refrigerate for at least 24 hours.

Prepare a mixture of the above herbs and spices, and stir in oil. Mix lightly to coat. Rub herb mixture into the leg of lamb with your hands.

Preheat oven to 325°. Place lamb in shallow roasting pan and bake uncovered for 2 to 2½ hours. If desired, onions and carrots may be added to the roasting pan at the end of one hour's time.

**May be converted to leftover salad. See "The Creative Leftover Roast" recipe.

"No Fail" Quiche Florentine

Servings: 6 to 8

Crust Ingredients:

    1½ cups whole wheat pastry flour
    ½ teaspoon sesame salt (optional)
    5 tablespoons cold butter
    3 to 4 tablespoons ice water

Crust Preparation:

Cut the butter into the flour and add sesame salt, using your hands or a pastry cutter, until the mixture looks like corn meal. Add water until dough can be gathered into a ball. Roll out on pastry cloth or between sheets of waxed paper. Place dough into 10" quiche pan. Cover with a sheet of waxed paper and weigh down with dried beans or uncooked rice. Bake in a preheated 375° oven for about 15 minutes. Remove paper and rice or beans and bake for another 5 minutes or until lightly browned. Cool on wire rack.

Filling Ingredients:

    2 cups cooked spinach, finely chopped
    3 cups sauce (recipe below)
    ½ teaspoon nutmeg
    1 whole egg
    2 egg yolks
    1 cup Swiss cheese, grated
    paprika

Filling Preparation:

Make sure spinach is free of moisture by mounding it in a double-folded piece of cheese cloth and squeezing it dry. Mix 2 cups of sauce with the spinach. Stir in 1 whole egg and the nutmeg. Spread mixture on the bottom of cooked crust. Stir the 2 egg yolks into the remaining cup of sauce and cover the spinach mixture. Add cheese as the final layer and finish by sprinkling paprika over the top. Bake in a 350° oven for about 20 to 25 minutes, until lightly browned and bubbly.

Sauce Ingredients:

    1 medium onion, finely chopped
    8 tablespoons butter
    2 tablespoons tamari soy sauce
    ½ teaspoon thyme
    dash of tabasco
    ½ cup whole wheat pastry flour
    1½ cups milk or light cream
    1½ cups white wine (vermouth is good)
    herbal salt to taste

Sauce Preparation:

Saute onion in butter until onion is tender, about 5 minutes. Add tamari soy sauce, thyme, tabasco, and flour to make a paste. Cook a minute or two longer. Pour the milk into the paste, add the wine, and stir with a wire whisk until smooth. Add a little more wine if a lighter sauce is desired. Add herbal salt to taste.

Savory Crepes

Servings: 10 to 12 filled crepes

FOLLOW SAME RECIPE UNDER "DESSERT CREPES" FOR PASTRY.

Filling Ingredients:

    1 medium onion, finely chopped
    ½ cup celery, finely chopped
    ¼ teaspoon each of dill, basil, thyme, and rosemary
    4 tablespoons butter
    1½ cups leftover lamb or beef, finely chopped

Filling Preparation:

Saute onion, celery, and herbs in butter for about 3 minutes, then add meat and heat thoroughly, stirring constantly. Divide the filling among the prepared crepes and spoon sauce over top.

Sauce Ingredients:

> 1 medium onion, finely chopped
> 8 tablespoons butter
> ½ cup whole wheat pastry flour
> 1 cup milk
> 2 cups beef broth
> herbal salt and thyme to taste

Sauce Preparation:

Saute the onion in butter until onion is tender, about 5 minutes. Add flour to make a paste and cook a minute or two longer. Pour the milk into the paste, add broth, stirring all the while with a wire whisk until smooth. Add herbal salt and thyme. Thin the sauce with a little vermouth if too thick. Makes about 3 cups of sauce.

Eggplant Rice Casserole

Servings: 4

Ingredients:

> 1½ pounds ground beef
> 1 large onion, chopped
> 4 cloves garlic, chopped
> 1 cup beef consomme
> ½ cup cooked brown rice
> 1½ cups fresh mushrooms, sliced
> 1 teaspoon sea salt
> 2 teaspoons cumin (or to taste)
> 1 teaspoon oregano
> 1 medium to large eggplant, sliced
> 3 medium tomatoes, sliced
> 1 cup grated Cheddar cheese

Preparation:

Mix together all ingredients except eggplant, tomatoes, and cheese. Cook in a frying pan over medium heat for about 5 minutes. Remove mixture from pan.

In a well-oiled casserole dish, arrange layers of meat/herb mix-

ture, eggplant slices, tomato slices, and cheese.
Bake in a 300° oven for about 2 hours. Serve hot.

Scallops With White Wine and Herbs* (low calorie)

Servings: 4

Ingredients:

>1 pound fresh or frozen scallops
>2 or 3 cloves garlic
>½ cup white wine
>1 tablespoon lemon juice
>parsley
>paprika

Preparation:

Place scallops in a shallow baking dish suitable for broiling. Crush garlic and add to wine in a small bowl. Stir in lemon juice. Sprinkle parsley and paprika over scallops, and pour wine mixture over all.
Broil for 10 minutes.

Variations:

This recipe is easily adaptable to most any kind of fish. With fillets, broil 7 minutes on each side.

Broiled Swordfish Steaks* (low calorie)

Servings: 4

Ingredients:

>1 two-pound swordfish steak, about 1½" thick
>½ cup fresh lemon juice
>1 teaspoon tarragon, finely chopped (or ½ teaspoon dried)
>2 teaspoons garlic, finely chopped
>2 tablespoons butter

Preparation:

Wash steak and dry with paper towels. Preheat oven to "Broil."

In a small saucepan, combine lemon juice, tarragon, butter, and garlic. Heat until butter is melted. Place steak in pan suitable for broiling that will allow juices to surround steak as it cooks. Cover the steak with butter mixture.

Broil 8 minutes per side, basting several times during process.

Serve steak at once on a heated platter. Arrange lemon wedge garnishes around steak in a ring formation.

Variations:

This same recipe can be adapted to your charcoal grill or habachi. Brush a tablespoon of oil over the grill and place the steak on the pre-heated surface. Brush both sides of the steak with the butter mixture and grill for about 8 minutes per side while it is 3" to 4" from heat source. The steak should be delicately browned and feel firm when prodded gently with a cooking utensil.

*Salmon Steaks Broiled With Herbs and Garlic** *(low calorie)*

Servings: 4

Ingredients:

4 salmon steaks about 1"thick
6 tablespoons butter
2 tablespoons shallots, chopped (or 3 tablespoons green onions, chopped)
3 tablespoons fresh parsley, finely chopped (or 2 tablespoons dried parsley)
1 to 1½ tablespoons garlic, finely chopped
1 or 2 lemons
few grains cayenne pepper

Preparation:

Preheat oven to "broil." Wash and dry salmon steaks with paper towels. Place in a pan suitable for broiling where steaks will rest in marinade sauce.

To make marinade, combine butter, shallots, parsley, garlic, lemon juice, cayenne pepper, and mix lightly, Spread over steaks and pour remainder into pan.

Broil 5 minutes per side and baste well. Turn again and baste, broiling another 6 to 8 minutes per side.

Transfer steaks to heated serving platter and cover with marinade and pan drippings. Garnish with lemon wedges, parsley and other greens.

Baked Oysters

Servings: 4

Ingredients:

2 tablespoons butter or olive oil
1 cup bread crumbs from preservative-free French or Italian bread
2 dozen fresh oysters
2 teaspoons garlic, finely chopped
3 tablespoons parsley, finely chopped (or 1¼ tablespoons dried)
4 tablespoons Parmesean cheese, freshly grated
2 tablespoons butter, in small chunks

Preparation:

This dish will serve four as a main course, or 6 to 8 as an **appetizer**.

Select an ovenproof shallow baking dish that is large enough to hold the oysters in one layer. Butter the dish well.

In a large skillet, melt 2 tablespoons butter or olive oil over moderate heat. Add bread crumbs and garlic, and toss together for about three minutes. Stir in parsley.

Spread 2/3's of this bread mixture into the bottom of the buttered baking dish. Arrange the oysters in a layer above this mixture. Spread the remaining bread mixture over the top. Sprinkle cheese to cover. Dot with butter chunks.

Bake in a moderate oven for 15 to 20 minutes, or until the crumb mixture is golden brown and the oysters are juicy and bubbling.

Stuffed Trout* *(low calorie)*

Servings: 4

Ingredients:

> 4 trout
> butter
> oil
> kelp salt (optional)
> 2 small carrots, shredded
> 1 meduim onion, finely chopped
> 2 stalks celery, finely chopped
> herbal salt, to taste (optional)
> cayenne pepper, to taste
> 4 tablespoons butter
> 1 teaspoon thyme

Preparation:

Saute the carrots, onions, and celery in 4 tablespoons butter, until soft, about 4 or 5 minutes. Sprinkle with herbal salt, if desired, thyme, and cayenne pepper.

Split and clean the trout. Stuff each one with a portion of the above mixture. Dot with butter and broil for 5 minutes. Use a touch of kelp salt when fish is removed from the broiler, if desired.

Wrap the fish in parchment paper. Oil the paper and place on buttered cookie sheet and bake at 425°. Allow 10 minutes cooking time per inch of thickness of fish, plus an additional 5 minutes for the heat to penetrate the parchment.

Linguini With White Clam Sauce

Servings: 4

Ingredients:

> 6 tablespoons olive oil
> 3 tablespoons garlic, finely chopped
> 1 cup clam broth
> ¼ cup dry white wine

3 doz. hard-shelled clams, shucked and minced (or 2 cans minced clams)
8 quarts water
1 pound pasta noodles (linguini or vermicelli page 171)
2 tablespoons fresh parsley, chopped (or 1 tablespoon dried)
sea salt (optional)
cayenne pepper

Preparation:

In a large heavy skillet, heat the oil making sure that it does not burn. Stir in garlic and cook for about one minute, then add clam broth and wine. Boil vigorously until liquid is reduced to about 3/4 of a cup. Remove from heat, set aside.

In a large kettle, boil 8 quarts water over high heat. Place pasta in boiling water and cook according to package instructions. Stir occasionally to prevent sticking. Transfer pasta to colander and drain thoroughly.

Return clam/wine sauce to heat and add fresh or minced clams. Cook over high heat, stirring constantly for about 2 minutes.

Arrange pasta on a platter and pour the sauce over it. Sprinkle with parsley and a few dashes of cayenne pepper, as desired.

Healthful Lasagna

Servings: 4 (with leftovers for reheating)

Ingredients:

12 to 14 strips lasagna noodles (pasta: see page 171)
3 tablespoons safflower oil
2 teaspoons sea salt (optional)
1 pound natural mozzarella cheese, sliced
1 cup grated Parmesean cheese
1½ cups natural cottage cheese
1½ cups natural ricotta cheese
8 oz. natural cream cheese
1 tablespoon grated onion
1 clove garlic, minced
1 tablespoon dill
herbal salt, to taste
2 tablespoons olive oil

Preparation:

Fill a large kettle three-quarters full of water. Add 3 tablespoons oil and 2 teaspoons of sea salt. Bring to a rolling boil. Add lasagna noodles and cook according to package instructions. Drain in a colander, rinse, and arrange on a paper towel to dry.

To make filling, rub the cottage cheese through a fine strainer. In an electric mixer, combine the cottage cheese, ricotta cheese, cream cheese, onion, garlic, and dill. Beat until light and fluffy. Add salt, if desired. Add olive oil and beat again. Put aside until final assembling of dish.

Sauce Ingredients:

>   2 16oz. cans tomato puree (unsalted)
>   4 tablespoons natural tomato paste
>   1 medium onion, finely chopped
>   2 cloves garlic, finely chopped
>   3 tablespoons olive oil
>   ½ cup water
>   1 cup Burgundy wine
>   4 tablespoons dried basil
>   2 tablespoons dried oregano
>   ¼ teaspoon cinnamon
>   drop honey

Sauce Preparation:

Saute the onions and garlic in olive oil. Cook for approximately 3 to 5 minutes. Add puree, paste, water, wine, basil, oregano, cinnamon, and honey to the onions and garlic. Let simmer for about one hour.

If desired, you may add about a pound of ground beef to make a meat sauce, or spaghetti sauce. Brown the ground beef in oil after adding garlic and onions, then add remaining ingredients.

FINAL ASSEMBLING:

Brush a shallow oblong pan with safflower oil. Place a layer of lasagna noodles on the bottom, then spread the cheese filling over top. Cover with a layer of sauce. Sprinkle some of the Parmesean cheese over top, then place slices of mozzarella over it. Continue to layer in this manner, ending with tomato sauce and a generous tier of cheese.

Bake in a 300° oven for about ½ an hour, or until thoroughly heated and bubbly.

Pizza

Servings: 3 ten-inch pizzas

Ingredients:

Dough Ingredients:

>*2 tablespoons dry yeast*
>*1¼ cups lukewarm water*
>*1 teaspoon honey (optional)*
>*1 cup soy flour*
>*2 cups rye flour (or whole wheat pastry flour)*
>*¾ teaspoon sea salt (optional)*
>*¼ cup olive oil*
>*corn meal to dust pans*

Sauce Ingredients:

>*1 cup onions, chopped*
>*4 cloves garlic, minced*
>*2 green peppers, diced*
>*2 tablespoons olive oil*
>*2 tablespoons safflower oil*
>*4 cups canned tomatoes (unsalted)*
>*1 small can tomato paste*
>*2 tablespoons oregano*
>*2 tablespoons basil*
>*1 tablespoon honey (optional)*
>*1 teaspoon sea salt (optional)*
>*2 cups mozzarella cheese, shredded*
>*½ cup Parmesean cheese, grated*

Dough Preparation:

Sprinkle dry yeast over surface of lukewarm water. Add honey (if desired), and let soak for 5 minutes.

Combine sifted soy flour, rye (or whole wheat) flour, and salt. Add to yeast mixture, Add oil and stir until dough is combined. Turn out onto floured board and knead until smooth and elastic. Place in an oiled bowl and cover with damp cloth. Let rise 1 to 2 hours in a warm place until doubled in size. Push dough down and knead briefly.

Divide dough into 3 balls of equal size and roll each one out to about an ⅛" thickness. Place on a baking sheet or pizza pan which has been dusted with corn meal. Make a rim around the pizza by pinching the crust into an edge. Preheat oven to 450°.

Sauce Preparation:

Saute onions, garlic, green pepper in mixed oils until tender. Add tomatoes, tomato paste, herbs, and seasonings. Simmer over low heat for about ½ an hour.

Top each pizza with about one cup of the tomato sauce, then ½ cup mozzarella cheese and 2 tablespoons Parmesean cheese.

Bake for about 15 minutes, or until browned and bubbly.

Stuffed Pork Chops

Servings: 4

Ingredients:

8 thin pork chops (or 4 thick ones with a pocket cut)
2 slices "day old" whole wheat bread
1 teaspoon dried thyme
½ teaspoon dried sage
4 tablespoons butter
1 medium onion, finely chopped
½ cup celery, finely chopped
½ cup orange juice
1 tablespoon honey
2 tablespoons tamari soy sauce
¼ teaspoon ground ginger

Preparation:

Crumble the bread and mix with thyme and sage. Melt butter in a frying pan and saute the onion and celery until lightly cooked (about 5 minutes). Add to bread mixture. Place 4 pork chops in baking pan, divide stuffing mixture among the four and top with remaining chops. (Or stuff the pockets of four thick chops). Mix together orange juice, honey, tamari soy sauce, and ginger. Pour over chops and bake in a pre-heated 350° oven for about 1 hour or until nicely browned.

Tasty Pot Roast*(low calorie)

Servings: 6 to 8

Ingredients:

>1 beef roast, 3 to 4 pounds
>1 teaspoon minced garlic (about 4 cloves)
>½ cup cider vinegar
>½ cup water
>1 teaspoon cumin
>½ teaspoon kelp seasoning
>½ teaspoon dried thyme
>3 bay leaves
>1 medium onion, sliced

Preparation:

Mix together garlic, vinegar, water, cumin, kelp seasoning, and thyme. After piercing holes all over the roast with a fork, pour the vinegar mixture over the meat, making sure some of the marinade seeps into the holes.

Let stand several hours, turning twice. Place meat in a covered roasting pan along with sliced onions and bay leaves. Cook in a preheated 325° oven for about 2 or 3 hours, or until tender.

Uncover last 30 minutes for browning. If desired, thicken cooking liquid with arrowroot (dissolve 1 teaspoon to one cup of cooking liquid in a small amount of cool water) or serve "as is" over the sliced meat.

Macaroni and Cheese

Servings: 4 to 6 generously

Ingredients:

>1 pound macaroni (pasta: see page 171)
>3 cups bechamel sauce (recipe below)
>4 oz. Parmesean cheese, grated
>1 pound mild cheddar cheese, coarsley grated

Preparation:

Having made the sauce (see below), cook the macaroni in boiling water according to package instructions. Combine the grated cheese and set aside. Butter a 2½ or 3 quart baking dish. As soon as macaroni is ready, drain and place ⅓ of it in the baking dish. Cover with one-third of the cheese and then one-third of the sauce. Make two more layers, sprinkling some extra cheese on the top. Put dish in a preheated 350° oven and bake for 15 to 20 minutes, or until lightly browned and bubbly.

Bechamel Sauce:

Saute 1 finely chopped, medium onion in 8 tablespoons butter until onion is tender (about 5 minutes). Add ½ cup pastry flour to make a paste and cook for a minute or two longer. Slowly pour 3 cups of hot milk into paste and stir with a wire whisk until smooth. Cook, stirring frequently, for about 15 to 20 minutes. Grate a bit of fresh nutmeg into sauce, to taste. Makes about 3½ cups.

Broiled Hamburgers (low calorie)*
Servings: 4

Ingredients:

> 1 pound ground beef
> 1 medium onion, chopped
> 1 teaspoon fresh garlic, minced
> 4 tablespoons fresh parsley, finely chopped
> 2 tablespoon tamari soy sauce
> ½ teaspoon kelp seasoning

Preparation:

Mix all ingredients and shape into patties. Broil 4 inches from flame until of desired doneness. Place on whole wheat hamburger buns. Add sliced tomato, sprouts, or lettuce, and any of the condiments that you prefer.

Variation:

Mix ½ lb. ground beef heart with hamburger for added nutrition. Or mix ¼ cup fresh wheat germ with hamburger.

The Creative Left-Over Roast* *(low calorie)*
Servings: 4 to 6

Ingredients:

> 1 cup cooked, left-over roast such as beef, lamb, or chicken, chopped
> ½ cup celery, finely chopped
> ½ medium onion, finely chopped
> 4 tablespoons fresh parsley, finely chopped
> 1 teaspoon dried dill
> ½ teaspoon dried thyme
> ¼ teaspoon dried tarragon
> 6 tablespoons plain yogurt
> ½ cup mayonnaise (if using beef, add a touch of horseradish to taste, if desired)

Preparation:

The meat can be put through a food processor, meat grinder, or chopped by hand. Combine meat, celery, onion, parsley, dill, thyme, and tarragon with yogurt and mayonnaise. Add a little more mayonnaise if mixture seems dry.

Spread on whole wheat or rye bread for a sandwich, adding sprouts for a special taste. Mixture can also be used as a salad. Use it to stuff tomatoes and surround it with sprouts or lettuce.

Breads, Pastry and Desserts

Whole Wheat Sourdough Bread Starter

Ingredients:

> ½ teaspoon dry yeast
> ¾ cup warm water
> ¾ cup whole wheat flour

Preparation:

Dissolve yeast in warm water. Stir in flour and mix well. Store in a clean glass jar or pottery container large enough to allow for some expansion. Place in a warm area for 18 to 24 hours. Stir Occasionally. At this point starter may be stored in refrigerator and used as a primary batter or starter.

To make batter for sourdough recipes, take out one cup of the starter and combine with 1 cup whole wheat flour and 1 cup lukewarm water. Mix well. There may be a few lumps, but these will dissolve in fermentation. Cover with a towel or plastic wrap and set in a warm location for several hours or overnight. Before adding additional ingredients, return at least ½ cup of the mixture to the starter storage container to replenish the stock.

Basic Whole Wheat Bread

Ingredients:

> 4 teaspoons dry yeast
> 1 cup lukewarm water
> 1 teaspoon honey
> ⅓ cup oil
> ¼ cup molasses
> 2 cups lukewarm water
> 1 tablespoon salt–optional
> 2 cups wheat germ
> 7 cups whole wheat flour
> 1 egg, beaten
> ¼ teaspoon water
> sesame seeds

Preparation:

Sprinkle yeast over top of lukewarm water, add honey. Leave to soak 5 to 10 minutes. Mix oil and molasses with 2 cups lukewarm water. Add salt and wheat germ. Add yeast mixture to oil/molasses/water mixture, stirring to combine.

Stir in 3½ cups flour, then stir in 3 remaining cups, mixing flour well. If necessary, add more flour.

Turn out onto a floured surface and knead in the remaining flour until dough is smooth and elastic. Knead for at least 10 minutes.

Place dough in an oiled bowl, turning once to coat the surface with oil to prevent drying. Cover with a damp cloth and let rise in a warm place until doubled in size—about 2 hours.

Punch dough down and let it rise for about 20 minutes. Knead another 5 minutes, then cut into two equal pieces and shape into two loaves. Place into well-oiled bread pans.

Brush tops with beaten egg and ¼ teaspoon water mixture. Sprinkle with sesame seeds. Let rise again until the loaves are high in pans—about 1½ hours.

Bake in a preheated 350° oven for about an hour, or until loaves sound hollow when thumped on the bottoms. Remove from pans and allow to cool before cutting.

Sourdough Applesauce Wheat Bread

Ingredients:

- 1 pkg. dry yeast
- ¼ cup warm water
- 1 cup sourdough starter
- ¼ cup safflower oil
- ½ cup raw sugar
- 1½ cups applesauce (without preservatives)
- 1 teaspoon salt (optional)
- 1 cup hot water
- 4 cups whole wheat flour
- ¼ teaspoon baking soda
- 2 to 3 cups unbleached flour
- melted butter

Preparation:

Mix together yeast and water. Set aside. In a large mixing bowl, combine sourdough starter, oil, sugar, applesauce, hot water, whole wheat flour, and baking soda. Mix well. Let rise for 10 minutes.

Blend in softened yeast mixture. Gradually add rest of flour as needed to make a moderately stiff dough. Turn onto floured surface and knead for 10 minutes, adding more flour when necessary. Place in a greased bowl, turning once to coat. Cover with a damp cloth. Set in a warm place free from drafts and allow to rise until doubled—about 2 hours.

Punch dough down and shape into two loaves. Place in oiled loaf pans. Cover, and let rise until doubled—about 1½ hours.

Bake in a preheated 350° oven for 35 to 45 minutes. Brush with melted butter.

No-Knead Whole Wheat Bread

Servings: 1 loaf

Ingredients:

    2 tablespoons honey
    ½ cup warm water
    1½ tablespoons dry yeast
    3¾ cups whole wheat flour
    1¼ cups warm water
    1 tablespoon salt (optional)

Preparation:

Stir honey and ½ cup warm water together. Mix in yeast and allow to stand until the mixture looks foamy.

In a large bowl, mix flour, salt, and yeast together. Slowly add the 1¼ cups warm water until dough is loose and sticky.

Grease a medium sized loaf pan with butter and add dough. Let rise for about one hour.

Bake 50 minutes in a 400° oven. Remove from pan and cool on a wire rack.

The New Health Hot Fudge Sauce

Servings: 1 cup

Ingredients:

    ⅓ cup honey
    6 ozs. carob chips
    1 teaspoon arrowroot
    ⅔ cup hot water
    ½ teaspoon pure vanilla

Preparation:

Combine the first four ingredients and simmer for 5 minutes while stirring constantly.

Remove from stove and add vanilla. Pour over ice cream and sprinkle with favorite nuts.

The Total Glow Carob Chip-Oatmeal Cookie

Servings: 24 to 30 cookies

Ingredients:

8 tablespoons softened butter
8 tablespoons honey
1 egg
1 teaspoon vanilla
2 teaspoons baking powder
1 cup whole wheat pastry flour
½ cup rolled oats
1 6oz. package carob chips
¾ cup coarsely chopped walnuts or pecans

Preparation:

In a large mixing bowl, combine butter and honey, and beat until light and fluffy. Beat in the egg and vanilla. Then add the baking powder and flour, beating in ¼ cup at a time. Fold in rolled oats, carob chips and walnuts or pecans.

Drop the batter by the rounded teaspoonful onto a buttered cookie sheet. Bake in a pre-heated 350° oven for about 12 to 15 minutes or until lightly browned. Cool on rack.

Yogurt Cheese Pie

Servings: 6 to 8

Ingredients:

1 pound cream cheese, softened at room temperature
1½ cups plain yogurt
6 tablespoons honey
1 teaspoon "lemon zest" (peel, cut very thin or grated)
¼ teaspoon ground cardamon

Preparation:

Whip cream cheese by hand or electric mixer until light and fluffy. Fold in yogurt, honey, lemon zest, and cardamon. Spread into a baked whole wheat pie shell (recipe below) and top with fresh fruit. A good topping is crushed pineapple or strawberries, sweetened to taste with honey.

Whole Wheat Pie Crust

Yield: one 9-inch pie shell

Ingredients:

> *1½ cups freshly ground whole wheat pastry flour*
> *½ teaspoon sesame salt (optional)*
> *5 tablespoons cold butter*
> *3 to 4 tablespoons ice water*

Preparation:

Cut the butter into the flour and salt, using your hands or a pastry cutter, until the mixture looks like corn meal. Add water until dough can be gathered into a ball.

Roll out on pastry cloth or between sheets of waxed paper. Place into pie pan, making a high edge around the outside. Place a piece of waxed paper in the shell and weight down with dried beans or uncooked rice. Bake in a pre-heated 400° oven for 10 minutes, then remove waxed paper and beans or rice. Continue to bake for about 5 minutes longer, or until brown. Allow shell to cool and use for any recipe calling for a baked pie shell.

Baked Peaches

Ingredients:

> *1 peach per person*
> *nutmeg*
> *cinnamon*
> *ginger*
> *brown sugar*
> *butter*

Preparation:

Preheat oven and lightly butter shallow baking pan.
Cut peaches into halves and discard pits. Arrange in pan, skin side

down. Place ½ teaspoon brown sugar in each peach, and ½ pat of butter. Sprinkle with spices.

Bake in a 350° oven for 15 minutes.

Remove peaches and pierce each one with a fork, being careful not to puncture the skin on the bottom. Return to oven and bake another 15 minutes.

Fruit, Nut, and Seed Candy

Servings: 32 pieces

Ingredients:

>½ cup dried apples
>1 cup dried apricots
>½ cup dried prunes, pitted
>½ cup raisins
>½ cup dates, pitted
>1 cup walnuts
>1 cup almonds
>½ cup sesame seeds
>½ cup sunflower seeds
>1 cup cashews, lighty toasted
>1 cup walnuts, ground
>1 teaspoon nutmeg, ground
>1 teaspoon cinnamon, ground
>½ teaspoon ginger, ground
>1 orange, peeled and quartered
>1 lemon, peeled and quartered

Preparation:

Prepare the dried fruit and nuts by either chopping finely by hand, a food processor, or hand grinder. If using a food processor, use the steel blade and process small amount of the dried fruits at a time.

Place mixture in a large bowl and add spices. Grind the sesame seeds, sunflower seeds, and cashews to a fine corn meal-like texture in a seed or coffee grinder, or blender.

Combine the fruit and nut mixture together in a large bowl. Place orange and lemon in a blender or food processor and process until they are a juicy pulp. Add this to the large bowl and mix with your hands.

After mixing thoroughly, form 1-inch balls and roll in ground walnuts. Store in refrigerator for up to 3 weeks.

High Protein Fudge

Ingredients:

>1 pound carob chips or flakes
>1 pound can peanut butter, sesame tahini, cashew butter, or almond honey
>2 tablespoons honey
>8 oz. English walnuts or black walnuts, chopped

Preparation:

In a saucepan, melt and blend together the first three ingredients over low heat. Stir continuously to prevent sticking and burning. When melted and smooth, remove from heat, add walnuts, and mix well.

Pour into a greased pan and decorate with whole walnuts. Chill in refrigerator for approximately 3 or 4 hours until fudge is firm for cutting. Cover tightly and store up to a week in the refrigerator.

Variations:

Coconut or raw dried fruits may be added.

Pie Crust Variations For Your Health

Coconut Pie Shell:

Ingredients:

>1 cup unsweetened coconut shreds
>½ cup fresh wheat germ
>2 tablespoons honey
>2 tablespoons oil

Preparation:

Preheat oven to 325°. Combine all ingredients and mix well. Press the mixture into a lightly oiled pie pan. Bake in the middle of the oven approximately 6 minutes, or until lightly browned. Cool before filling.

Standard Healthy Pie Crust Mix:

Ingredients:

⅓ cup sesame seeds, freshly ground
⅓ cup almonds, freshly ground
⅓ cup sunflower seeds, freshly ground
2 tablespoons fresh wheat germ
½ teaspoon cinnamon
½ teaspoon nutmeg
⅓ cup soft butter -or- ⅓ cup oil and 1 tablespoon honey

Preparation:

Mix all ingredients until crumbly and press into a lightly oiled pie plate. Bake about 15 minutes in a moderate oven until lightly browned.

Carrot Cake

Ingredients:

1 cup softened butter
1¼ cups honey
4 eggs
1½ cups grated carrots
1 cup whole wheat pastry flour
1 cup unbleached flour
3 teaspoons baking powder
1 teaspoon cinnamon
½ teaspoon nutmeg
½ teaspoon salt (optional)
⅔ cup nuts, coarsely chopped

Preparation:

Cream together butter and honey. Beat in eggs one at a time. Add carrots and blend well.

Sift together flours, baking powder, spices, and salt. Add to carrot mixture along with water. Add nuts and beat batter well.

Pour into 2 buttered layer cake pans and bake in a preheated 350° oven for 25 to 30 minutes or until firm in the middle. Cool and frost with cream cheese and honey frosting.

Cream Cheese and Honey Frosting:

Soften cream cheese (about 12 oz) and sweeten with as much honey as desired.

Cheese Cake

Ingredients:

Crust:

1 cup wheat germ
4 tablespoons oil
1 tablespoon honey
½ teaspoon cinnamon

Combine ingredients and pat into spring form pan, covering bottom and bringing up on the sides about 1½ inches.

Filling:

¼ cup arrowroot powder
1 cup yogurt
1 pound cottage cheese
rind of one lemon, grated
1 tablespoon lemon juice
¼ teaspoon salt (optional)
½ cup honey
2 teaspoons vanilla extract
4 eggs, separated

Preparation:

In a blender, blend arrowroot and yogurt until arrowroot is dissolved. Add cottage cheese and blend until smooth. Add lemon rind, juice, salt, honey, vanilla, and blend to combine well.

Beat egg yolks in a mixing bowl until thick and lemon-colored. Add to the cheese mixture and mix well. Beat egg whites until stiff but not dry. Fold into cheese mixture and pour into prepared pan.

Bake in a preheated 350° oven for about an hour. When cake is cool, loosen sides of spring form pan and remove from cake. Refrigerate cake for a few hours or overnight before serving.

Carob Cake

Ingredients:

>*1 cup whole wheat pastry flour*
>*½ cup carob powder*
>*3 teaspoons baking powder*
>*½ teaspoon salt (optional)*
>*⅔ cup finely chopped nuts*
>*2 eggs*
>*1 cup milk*
>*1 cup honey*
>*¼ cup oil*

Preparation:

Combine flour, carob powder, baking powder, and salt. Separate eggs. Combine yolks, milk, honey, and oil. Add this to flour mixture and beat well. Stir in nuts.

Beat egg whites until stiff and fold into batter. Turn into a well-oiled 8-inch square baking pan and bake in a preheated 350° oven for 50 **to** 60 minutes, or until toothpick comes out clean.

Dessert Crepes

Servings: 10–12 crepes

Ingredients:

>*8 tablespoons whole wheat pastry flour*
>*dash of sea salt (optional)*
>*1 whole egg*
>*yolk of one egg*
>*3 tablespoons safflower oil*
>*¾ cup milk*
>*additional safflower oil for pan*

Preparation:

In a small bowl, beat together the flour, optional salt, whole egg, egg yolk and safflower oil. Add additional milk to give the batter the consistency of light cream. Cover the bowl with plastic wrap and let it sit in the refrigerator for at least 30 minutes or longer.

Prepare crepes according to your crepe pan's directions, using the additional safflower oil.

Fillings can be prepared with fresh fruits, fruit concentrates, and cottage cheese or ricotta cheese sweetened with honey. Honey-sweetened ice cream with a carob sauce is an excellent choice.

*Frozen Fruit Delight** (low calorie)

Servings: 4

Ingredients:

    2 frozen bananas, peeled
    1 frozen peach**
    1 frozen apple (do not seed)**
    1 frozen pear (do not seed)**
    1 small can pineapple tidbits (emptied into a plastic sandwich bag and frozen)
    3 oz. tofu (optional)
    4 eggs (optional)

Preparation:

Place all ingredients in a blender or food processor, and whip until well blended.

Serve in a brandy snifter or dessert dish, with spoons.

**Freeze in quarter slices with skin in tact

Carob Chip Cookies

Servings: 24 to 30 cookies

Ingredients:

    8   tablespoons softened butter
    8   tablespoons honey

1 teaspoon vanilla
1 egg
2 teaspoons baking powder
1½ cups whole wheat pastry flour
1 6oz. package carob chips
¾ cup coarsley chopped walnuts

Preparation:

In a large mixing bowl, combine butter and honey, beating until light and fluffy. Beat in the vanilla and egg. Add baking powder and flour, beating in ¼ cup at a time. Fold in carob chips and walnuts.

Drop the batter by rounded teaspoonsful onto a buttered cookie sheet. Bake in a pre-heated 350° oven for about 12 minutes, or until lightly browned.

Carob Brownies

Servings: 16 pieces

Ingredients:

4 tablespoons carob powder
6 tablespoons butter, melted
½ cup honey
2 eggs, well beaten
1 cup whole wheat pastry flour
½ teaspoon baking powder
1 teaspoon vanilla
1 cup coarsley chopped walnuts

Preparation:

Add carob powder to melted butter. It may look a little grainy, but will bake out. Beat the eggs until light and gradually add the honey, beating thoroughly. Blend in the carob mixture. Combine flour and baking powder and sift twice. Mix flour and carob mixture, blending in several tablespoons at a time. Pour in batter and bake in a pre-heated 350° oven for 30 minutes, or until a knife inserted in the middle comes out clean. Cool, then cut into 2-inch squares.

Total Glow Party Buffet Menu

Assorted fresh, raw vegetables with Dips*
(Choose 2 or 3 different dips from recipes provided, and 4 to 6 vegetables from list, or more if in season. Wash and slice vegetables just before serving.)
>Varieties:
>>Carrots, green peppers, cucumbers, yellow squash, broccoli, cauliflower, zucchini, green beans, asparagus, cherry tomatoes, spring onions, celery

Assorted Cheese Tray with Crackers
>(Select as many cheeses as desired. Choose several types of crackers that are made without preservatives and salt-free).
>>*Varieties of cheese:*
>>>Gruyere, Gouda, Jarlesberg, Sharp Cheddar, Brie, Bleu Cheese, Tilsit, Muenster

Marianated Mushrooms (recipe included)*
Hot Clam Squares (recipe included)
Bar-B-Que Beef with Rolls (beef recipe included, make your own rolls from recipes, or choose preservative-free brand)
Hot Chicken Salad (recipe included)*
Kidney Bean Salad with Cheese and Apples (recipe included)
Variation Fruit Salad (recipe included)*
Carob-chip Oatmeal Cookies (recipe included)

Hot Clam Squares
Servings: 32 squares

Ingredients:

>2 tablespoons chopped onion
>1 tablespoon butter
>1½ tablespoons unbleached flour
>1 teaspoon tamari soy sauce
>1 to 2 tablespoons crushed clove garlic
>1 7oz. can minced clams with juice
>8 slices bread (preservative-free)

Preparation:

Melt butter in small saucepan over medium heat, add onion and cook until onions are clear, stirring occasionally for two to three minutes. Blend in flour and stir until smooth.

Add remaining ingredients and cook over low heat until thick (about five to seven minutes). Cool in refrigerator for about 10 minutes.

Meanwhile, cut off crusts on each slice of bread and divide slices into four equal squares.

Spread each square with the cooled clam mixture. Bake at 425° for eight to ten minutes. Serve hot.

Can be prepared ahead of time and frozen or kept in refrigerator until ready to use.

Bar-B-Q Beef* *(low calorie)*
Serves: Main course—10 to 12 people
Party dish—18 to 20 people

Ingredients:

3½ to 4 pound pot roast or chuck roast
1 8oz. can of beer
1 large onion, chopped
2 or 3 cloves garlic, chopped
3 small bottles ketchup (made with honey)
¼ cup tamari soy sauce
¼ cup apple cider vinegar
2 teaspoons chili powder
2 teaspoons turbingo sugar or honey
2 teaspoons dry mustard

Preparation:

Trim fat off pot roast and place in large pot suitable for oven. Add onion and garlic to meat and pour beer over all. Cook in oven at 350° for 3½ to 4 hours.

After meat has cooked, cool in refrigerator several hours. Shred beef into long, thin pieces by cutting off chunks of meat and pulling them apart with fingers. (If meat does not pull apart easily, it has not cooked long enough. Return to oven for another 30 to 45 minutes.

Place the shredded beef in a large pot and drain liquid from roasting pan into shredded beef. Add all ingredients and cook over medium heat stirring occasionally. When mixture begins to boil, turn heat to simmer. Scrape bottom of pan to avoid burning.

Simmer at least an hour. Added time will enhance the flavor.

Mixture may be prepared ahead of time and frozen for several weeks.

Serve with rolls.

Hot Chicken Salad* *(low calorie)*

Servings: Main course—4 to 6 people
Party dish—10 to 12 people

Ingredients:

>1½ to 2 cups cooked chicken, cut into small pieces
>1 cup blender mayonnaise (recipe preceding)
>2 stalks celery, chopped
>1 medium onion, chopped
>½ cup slivered almonds
>1 teaspoon thyme // 1 teaspoon parsley
>¼ teaspoon sea salt (optional–if desired)

Preparation:

Place chicken in large mixing bowl with celery, onions, almonds, mayonnaise, parsley, and thyme. Mix thoroughly. Place in an oblong casserole dish and bake at 350° for 30 to 45 minutes. Serve hot.

This dish can be prepared ahead of time and refrigerated. Allow 20 minutes extra cooking time after refrigeration. Left over salad is also good cold, by itself or in a sandwich.

Kidney Bean Salad With Cheese and Apples

Servings: 6 to 8

Ingredients:

>1 24oz. can red kidney beans
>1 cup mayonnaise
>1 small onion chopped
>1 stalk celery, chopped
>1 large apple, chopped
>1 cup cheddar cheese, cubed

Preparation:

Drain kidney beans and place in large mixing bowl. Add remaining ingredients and mix thoroughly. Refrigerate one to two hours before serving.

Variation Fruit Salad* (low calorie)
Servings: 10 to 12

Ingredients:

>   (Varies with fruits in season)
>
>   1 or 2 bananas, sliced
>   1 16oz. can pineapple chunks (water-pack)
>   1 sm. package shredded coconut
>   1 16oz. carton plain yogurt (or more if needed depending on amount of fruit)
>   ¼ to ½ cup honey (to taste)
>   Select two or more kinds of fruit from list below:

Apples, Oranges, Pears, Peaches, Melon, Strawberries, Blueberries, Apricots

Preparation:

Mix all ingredients lightly and chill in refrigerator for at least and hour before serving.

Seven Day Menu Plan

The following seven-day meal plan is an example of the way in which you can schedule your meals, if you prefer to do it that way. Some find it easier to do their weekly shopping if they have planned in advance what they will serve. Others like to be more spontaneous. It's up to you; whichever you prefer. However, planning ahead will result in saving both time and money, but, like any habit, will take some time to develop. It can also make cooking alot more fun.

First Day

Breakfast: 1 6oz. glass of juice
Scrambled Eggs (recipe included)
1 slice whole wheat toast (or equivalent) (recipe incl.)
Preservative-free jelly (optional)
Lunch: Tuna Salad Sandwich (recipe included)
Carob-chip Oatmeal Cookies (recipe included)
Milk/Juice/Herbal Tea
Dinner: Tasty Pot Roast (recipe included)
Steamed Carrots & Potatoes (instructions included)
Garden Salad (Use greens and vegetables in season)
Honey Ice Cream with Hot Fudge Sauce (recipe included)

Second Day

Breakfast: 1 6oz. glass of juice (or slice of melon)
Homemade Cereal (recipe included)
Milk/Herbal Tea/Coffee Substitute such as Mellow Roast
Lunch: Vegetarian Carrot Sandwich/Salad (recipe included)
Fresh Fruit (or yogurt)
Dinner: Lemon Tarragon Chicken (recipe included)
Pineapple Coleslaw (recipe included)
Stewed Eggplant (or Roasted Corn) (recipes included)
Carob Cake (recipe included)

Third Day

Breakfast: 1 6oz. glass of juice
Whole Wheat Pancakes (recipe included)

Introduction to the Recipes 249

              Homemade Sausage (recipe included)
              Honey
Lunch: Tossed Salad
              Cold Lemon Tarragon Chicken (left-over from previous night)
              Carob Cake (left-over from previous night)
Dinner: Gazpacho Soup (recipe included)
              Creative Left-over Roast (recipe included)
              Rye Bread or Sour Dough Bread (recipes included)
              Steamed Green Beans (instructions included)
              Baked Peaches (recipe included) or fresh fruit (optional)

Fourth Day

Breakfast: 1 6oz. glass of juice (or grapefruit half)
              Healthy Egg Muffin (recipe included)
              Milk/Herbal Tea/Coffee Substitute
Lunch: Broiled Hamburger (recipe included) or nitrate-free lunchmeat sandwich
              Fresh fruit (or yogurt)
Dinner: Scallops or Fish Fillets with White Wine and Herbs (recipe included)
              Steamed Asparagus or Broccoli (instructions included)
              Raw Mushrooms with Herbs Salad (recipe included)
              Cheese Cake (recipe included) (optional)

Fifth Day (especially for busy days)

Breakfast: Nutrition Drink (recipe included)
Lunch: Peanut Butter and Jelly Sandwich (recipe included)
              Fresh Fruit
Dinner: Broiled Chicken Italian (recipe included)
              Steamed Yellow Squash (instructions included)
              Sweet & Sour Marianated Cucumbers & Onion Salad (recipe included)
              Honey Ice Cream with Fresh Fruit or Nuts

Sixth Day

Breakfast: 1 6oz. glass of juice
              Basic Omelet with Cheese (recipe included)

	English Muffin with jelly (preservative-free)
Lunch:	Hearty Vegetable Soup (recipe included)
	Homemade Bread (recipes included)**
Dinner:	Baked Oyster Appetizer (recipe included)
	Healthful Lasagna (recipe included)***
	Salad Greens (in season)
	Dessert Crepes with Fruit and Honey Filling (recipe included)

Seventh Day

Use up left-overs for lunch, and enjoy a nice dinner in a restaurant.

**Always refrigerate for following week's use.
***Make extra sauce, freeze for spaghetti later on in week

Supplemental Readings

Converting your recipes

The following is an illustration of how you might convert two ordinary recipes into healthful ones using only natural ingredients. They are recipes for chocolate-chip cookies (converting from chocolate and sugar to carob and honey) and for brownies (converting the same ingredients).

Making these conversions is really not difficult, and with a little imagination, most any ordinary cookbook recipe may be converted in this fashion.

Converting this recipe to more healthful ingredients, the list would read like this:

Basic Chocolate Chip Cookies

Yield: 24 to 30 Cookies

Ingredients:
- 8 tablespoons softened butter or margarine
- 6 tablespoons granulated sugar
- 6 tablespoons dark brown sugar
- ½ teaspoon salt
- 1 teaspoon vanilla flavoring
- 1 egg
- ½ teaspoon baking soda
- 1 cup white flour
- 1 6 oz. package chocolate chips
- ¾ cup coarsley chopped walnuts

Carob Chip Cookies

Yield: 24 to 30 Cookies

Ingredients:
- 8 tablespoons softened butter
- 8 tablespoons honey
- 1 teaspoon natural vanilla
- 1 egg
- 2 teaspoons baking powder
- 1½ cups whole wheat pastry flour
- 1 6 oz. package carob chips (sweetened)
- ¾ cup coarsley chopped walnuts

Preparation for Carob Chip Cookies:

In a large mixing bowl, combine butter and honey, beating until light and fluffy. Beat in vanilla and egg, then add baking powder and flour, beating in ¼ cup at a time. Fold in carob chips and walnuts.

Drop the batter by rounded teaspoonsful onto a buttered cookie sheet. Bake in preheated 350° oven for about 12 minutes, or until lightly browned.

Converting this recipe to more healthful ingredients, the list would read like this:

Basic Brownies	Carob Brownies
Yield: 16 pieces	Yield: 16 pieces
Ingredients:	Ingredients:
2 squares unsweetened chocolate	4 tablespoons carob powder
8 tablespoons softened butter or margarine	6 tablespoons butter, melted
1 cup sugar	½ cup honey
2 eggs	2 eggs, well beaten
½ cup white flour	1 cup whole wheat pastry flour
½ teaspoon baking powder	½ teaspoon baking powder
½ teaspoon salt	
1 teaspoon vanilla flavoring	1 teaspoon natural vanilla
1 cup coarsley chopped walnuts	1 cup coarsley chopped walnuts

Preparation for Carob Brownies:

Add carob powder to the melted butter (grainy texture will bake out). Beat the eggs until light and gradually add honey, beating thoroughly. Blend in carob/butter mixture. Combine flour and baking powder and sift twice. Mix flour into carob mixture, blending in several tablespoons at a time. Fold in nuts and vanilla.

Lightly butter an eight-inch square pan, pour in the batter and bake in a preheated 350° oven for 30 minutes, or until a knife inserted in the middle comes out clean.

Cool, then cut into 2-inch squares.

How to Grow Your Own Sprouts

You could have a continuous garden of fresh salad supplies right in your kitchen. Sprouts are a wonderful vegetable, carrying all the vitamins and minerals found in the beans or grains from which they are grown, but only a fraction of the calories. They can grow in any climate, they require neither sun nor soil, and the nutritive value will rival tomatoes in Vitamin C. Sprouts retain the B-Complex vitamins present in the original seed, and a large amount of Vitamin A.

There is quite a variety of seeds that can be sprouted. Among the more common ones are alfalfa, mung beans, soy beans, adjuki beans, chia, fenugreek, lentil, and wheat. The methods of sprouting are also varied, but perhaps the most common is to use a wide-mouth glass jar with the opening covered by a piece of cheese cloth or similar open-weave fabric. Secure the cloth with a rubber band.

The technique is as follows:

1. Rinse the seeds thoroughly. A strainer or sieve can be used. Or you may put the seeds directly into the jar, secure the cheese cloth, fill the jar with water, swish, and drain.

2. Cover the seeds with additional water and allow to soak overnight.

3. In the morning, pour off the soaking water (which can later be used as a base for soup).

4. Tilt the jar to allow for additional draining and place in a dark cupboard.

5. Rinse the seeds several times a day. A few seeds, such as soybean, need to be rinsed about 4 to 6 times daily depending on the temperature.

6. By the second day you should be seeing tiny sprouts. Alfalfa seeds are usually ready to eat in 3 to 4 days. Bigger seeds take longer. Let them grow to the desired size, then rinse thoroughly and store in glass jars in the refrigerator or freezer.

Sprouts can be eaten raw or used in cooked dishes such as stir-fried vegetables. You might try stirring some sprouts into your next batch of muffins or other quick bread. They are also delicious in egg dishes, like omelettes and quiches. The possibilities are endless!

Some Helpful Household Utensils

Throughout the food sections, I have mentioned several appliances and utensils which you may be interested in purchasing to complete your health food kitchen. Following is a list of the major appliances, what they do, and a general price range.

Juicer: Raw juices are rich in vitamins, minerals, trace elements, enzymes, and natural sugar, thereby making the juicer one of the most important items in the kitchen. They range in price and quality from $60 to $250, and can be purchased from a health food store, department store, discount house, or catalog.

Blender: A blender is a useful item, especially when preparing nutritious milkshakes, fruit drinks, salad dressings, etc. It can be purchased from any of the above mentioned sources for as little as $15 to $40.

Seed Mill: A small electric seed mill is handy to have for grinding up seeds and nuts, and small amounts of grains for cereals. Their price range is normally from $13 to $30.

Yogurt Maker: This appliance takes the guess work out of making your own fresh yogurt. There are several different brand names on the market and range in price from about $10 to $17.

Food Processor: The food processor is a dream machine that speeds up such mundane procedures as chopping and mincing. It's a great asset to any kitchen and in addition to chopping, it will grate, mince, slice, puree, and make pie and bread dough in a very rapid manner. There is a great deal of competition among food processors, and prices range from $60 to $230.

Flour Mill: This appliance is essential if you are grinding your own flour, but it is expensive. The price can range from $160 to $275. If this is beyond your budget, perhaps a cooperative venture with neighbors would be in order.

Steamers: There are several vegetable steamers on the market, the most popular being a wire basket which sells for about $4. Pottery steamers can also be had for as much as $25.

SELECTED BIBLIOGRAPHY

Airola, Paavo, Ph.D., N.D. *Are You Confused?* Phoenix: Health Plus Publishers, 1971.
Airola, Paavo, Ph.D., N.D. *Cancer, The Total Approach.* Phoenix: Health Plus Publishers, 1972.
Airola, Paavo, Ph.D., N.D. *How to Get Well.* Phoenix: Health Plus Publishers, 1974.
Barnes, Broda O. and Galton, Lawrence. *Hypo-thyroidism: The Unsuspected Illness.* New York: Thomas Y. Crowell Co., 1976.
Beecher, Willard and Beecher, Margarite. *Beyond Success and Failure.* New York: Simon & Schuster, 1966.
Benson, Herbert, M.D. *The Relaxation Response.* New York: William Morrow and Co., Inc., 1975.
Bernstein, Douglas A. and Borkovec, Thomas D. *Progressive Relaxation Training.* Champaign, Illinois: Research Press, 1973.
Carrington, Patricia, Ph.D. *Freedom in Meditation.* New York: Doubleday & Co., 1977.
Cooper, Kenneth H., M.D. *Aerobics.* New York: Bantam Books, 1968.
Cooper, Kenneth H., M.D. and Cooper, Mildred. *Aerobics for Women.* New York: Bantam Books, 1972.
Dufty, William. *Sugar Blues.* New York: Warner Books, 1975.
Fixx, James F. *The Complete Book of Running.* New York: Random House, 1977.
Fredericks, Carlton, Ph.D. *Breast Cancer: A Nutritional Approach.* New York: Grosset and Dunlap Publishers, 1977.
Fredericks, Carlton, Ph.D. *Look Younger, Feel Healthier.* New York: Grosset and Dunlap Publishers, 1972.
Hittleman, Richard. *Guide to Yoga Meditation.* New York: Bantam Books, 1977.
Hittleman, Richard. *Yoga: The 8 Steps to Health and Peace.* New York: Bantam Books, 1976.
Kelley, William Donald, B.A., D.D.A., M.S., F.I.C.A.N. *One Answer to Cancer.* Beverly Hills: The Kelley Foundation, 1969.
Krupp, Marcus A., Chatton, Milton J., and Margen, Sheldon. *Current Diagnosis and Treatment.* Los Altos, California: Lange Medical Publications, 1971.
Levy, Juliette de Bairacli. *The Complete Herbal Book for the Dog.* New York: Arco Publishing Co., Inc., 1971.
Nittler, Alan, M.D. *A New Breed of Doctor.* New York: Pyramid Publications, 1974.
Passwater, Richard A. *Supernutrition.* New York: The Dial Press, 1975.
Rodale, J.I. and Staff. *The Complete Book of Minerals for Health.* Emmaus, Pennsylvania: Rodale Books, Inc., 1976.

Thorn, George W., Adams, Richard D., Branuwald, Eugene, Isselbacher, Kurt J., and Petersdorf, Robert G., editors. *Harrison's Principles of Internal Medicine* (revised edition). New York: McGraw Hill Book Company, 1977.
Ubell, Earl. *How to Save Your Life.* New York: Harcourt Brace Jovanovich, Inc., 1976.
Williams, Roger J., M.D. *Nutrition Against Disease.* New York: Pittman Publishing Corp., 1971.
Williams, Roger J., M.D. *The Wonderful World Within You.* New York: Bantam Books, Inc., 1977.
Williams, Roger J., M.D. *You are Extraordinary.* New York: Pittman Publishing Corp., 1967.

SUGGESTED READINGS

Aerobics, Kenneth H. Cooper, M.D.
  Bantam Books, Inc.
  666 Fifth Avenue
  New York, NY 10019
Aerobics for Women, Kenneth H. and Mildred Cooper.
  Bantam Books, Inc.
  666 Fifth Avenue
  New York, NY 10019
Are You Confused?, Paavo Airola, Ph.D., N.D.
  Health Plus Publishers
  P. O. Box 22001
  Phoenix, AZ 85028
Breast Cancer: A Nutritional Approach, Carlton Fredericks, Ph.D.
  Grosset and Dunlap, Publishers
  51 Madison Avenue
  New York, NY 10010
Cancer, The Total Approach, Paavo Airola, Ph.D., N.D.
  Health Plus Publishers
  P.O. Box 22001
  Phoenix, AZ 85028
The Complete Book of Minerals for Health, J. I. Rodale and Staff
  Rodale Books, Inc.
  Emmaus, PA 18049
The Complete Book of Running, James F. Fixx
  Random House, Inc.
  201 East 50th St.
  New York, NY 10022
How to Get Well, Paavo Airola, Ph.D., N.D.
  Health Plus Publishers
  P. O. Box 22001
  Phoenix, AZ 85028
Hypothyroidism: The Unsuspected Illness, Broda O. Barnes, M.D., and Lawrence Galton
  Thomas Y. Crowell Co.
  666 Fifth Avenue
  New York, NY 10019
Look Younger, Feel Healthier, Carlton Fredericks, Ph.D.
  Grosset and Dunlap, Publishers
  51 Madison Avenue
  New York, NY 10010
The New Aerobics, Kenneth H. Cooper, M.D.
  Bantam Books, Inc.
  666 Fifth Avenue
  New York, NY 10019

A New Breed of Doctor, Alan Nittler, M.D.
   Pyramid Publications
   919 Third Avenue
   New York, NY 10022

Nutrition Against Disease, Roger J. Williams, M.D.
   Pittman Publishing Corp.
   6 East 43rd Street
   New York, NY 10017

One Answer to Cancer, William Donald Kelley, B.A., D.D.S., M.S., F.I.C.A.N.
   The Kelley Foundation
   The International Assn. of Cancer Victims and Friends, Inc.
   Box 3718
   Beverly Hills, CA 90212

Sugar Blues, William Dufty
   Warner Books, Inc.
   75 Rockefeller Plaza
   New York, NY 10019

Supernutrition, Richard A. Passwater
   The Dial Press
   1 Dag Hammarskjold Plaza
   New York, NY 10017

The Wonderful World Within You, Roger J. Williams, M.D.
   Bantam Books, Inc.
   666 Fifth Avenue
   New York, NY 10019

You Are Extraordinary, Roger J. Williams, M.D.
   Pyramid Publications
   919 Third Avenue
   New York, NY 10022

COOKBOOKS:

The Delicious World of Raw Food, Mary Louise Lau
   Rawson Associates, Publishers, Inc.
   630 Third Avenue
   New York, NY 10017

The New York Times Natural Foods Cookbook, Jean Hewitt
   Quadrangle Books, Inc.
   330 Madison Avenue
   New York, NY 10017

**The Rodale Cookbook,* Nancy Albright
   Rodale Press, Book Division
   Emmaus, PA 18049

*Good for the beginner.

Sprouts to Grow and Eat, Esther Munroe
    Stephen Greene Press
    Box 1000
    Brattleboro, VT 05301
Tassajara Cooking, Zen Center
    Shambhala Publications, Inc.
    2045 Francisco Street
    Berkeley, CA 94709
**The Dione Lucas Book of Natural French Cooking,* Marion Gorman and
    Felipe P. de Alba
    E. P. Dutton & Co., Inc.
    201 Park Avenue, South
    New York, NY 10003

**For the gourmet.

Index

Additives/Preservatives, 3, 6, 10, 93-94, 108, 120, 123
Aerobic exercise, 86
Aging, 107
Airola, Paavo, Ph.D., N.D., 109, 135, 142, 146
Alcoholism, 6
Alpha brain wave level, 43, 52, 53
American Cancer Society, 124-125
Anxiety, 35, 39
Aremueller, H., Dr., 143
Aristotle, 19
Artherosclerosis, 5, 60
Arthritis, xv, 39
Assertiveness, 36
Athletes, 59
Australian Medical Journal, 121

Backaches, xv, 39
Baking powder, 112
Bee pollen, 112
Benson, Herbert, 43
Beta brain wave level, 43
BHT/BHA, 121
Blood lactate level, 45
Bowling, 57
Brain waves, 43
Bread, 110, 121, 143
Brosse, Therese, 43

Cancer, xv, 3, 11, 124, 140
Carbohydrates, 99, 116

Carob, 110, 166
Cereals, 111
Childbirth, 59
Children, 123, 139, 175
Chocolate, 110
Coffee, 170
Cooking, 108
Cookware, 172
Cooper, Dr. Theodore, 4
Condiments, 112
Consumer Reports, 117
Controlled breathing, 48
Costill, Dr. David, 5
Crackers, 110
Crash diets, 58
Crisis medicine, 136
Criticism, 33
Cycling, 82

Dancing, 58
Davis, Adele, 23
Delta brain wave level, 43
Detoxification organs, 122, 129, 144
Diabetes/diabetic, 51, 107, 116
Diet Awareness Questionnaire, 105
Dieticians, 136
Dieting/weight reduction, 3, 34, 107
Diverticulosis, xv
Dreaming/dreams, 44
Drug addiction/dependence, 6
Dufty, William, 115

Index

Eggs, 112
Environmental Protection Agency, 109, 156
Exercise, 14, 15, 54, 57, 162
Expectations, 50
Extrasensory perception, 44, 52

Faddism, 128
F.D.A., 9, 94, 127
Fiengold, Benjamin F., 3
Fiber, 108, 141
"Fight or flight" reaction, 2
Flour, 110
Fluoridation, 23
Focus (in meditation), 20, 54
Fredericks, Carlton, 23, 121
Fruits, 111

Golf, 57
Guidelines, 167
Guilt, 16, 94

Habits, 34
Harvard University, 43
Headaches, xv, 6, 39, 41
Health Barometer, 183
Health foods, xv, 108, 128, 162, 175
Health Policy, 164
Health Questionnaire, 27-28
Healthview Newsletter, 142
Heart disease, xv, 3, 60
Height/weight charts, 96, 97, 98
Herbs, 112
Hereditary, 57, 92
Holidays, 25
Homemakers, 20
Horseback riding, 57
Hostility, 54
Human integration, 1
Hypertension/high blood pressure, 6, 39, 41, 53, 60
Hypothyroidism, 154

Ice cream, ingredients in, 122
Illustrative method of meditation, 48

Insecticides/Pesticides, 125
Insight, 21, 44
Insomnia, 6
Insulin, 115
Interruptions during meditation, 55
Ivy, A.C., 143

Jams/jellies, 110
Jogging, 16, 37, 58, 86, 97
Juices, 109, 169
Junk food, 24, 93, 128

Kelley, William D., M.D., 99, 135
Kiphuth, Delaney, 5

Labeling laws, 116
Laetrile, 23
Legumes, 111, 172
Le Shan, Lawrence, 32, 39
Let's Live Magazine, 115, 142
Lewis, Howard R. and Martha E., 32
Life expectancy, 10
Liver, 134, 143
Longfellow, Henry Wadsworth, 21
"Looking glass self" concept, 33
"Lotus" position, 49
Love terms, 26
Lung cancer, xv

Mantra, 20, 49
Massage, 132
Mayonnaise, 111
McGovern, George, 3
Meat/Poultry/Fish, 112
Medical schools, 4, 135
Meditation, 7, 14, 19, 39, 173-174
Megavitamin therapy, 23
Memory, 44, 45
Metabolic rate/metabolism, 45, 99, 142
"Middle aged spread", 57
Mind-over-matter concept, 44
Moderation, 95, 134

Index

National Cancer Institute, 4, 141, 156
National Health Federation Newsletter, 158
Natural foods, xv, 109, 128, 162, 175
Negative slogans, 3
Newsweek, 141
Nitrates/Nitrites, 109, 158
Non-foods, 93
Nutrition, 14, 22
Nuts/grains, 111

Obesity/overweight, 5, 17, 34, 55, 60, 141
Oil, 109, 143
Organic produce, 127
Organs of detoxification, 122, 129, 144
Oxygen consumption, 45

Pasta, 110, 171
Pauling, Linnus, 23
Penicillin, 9
Pepper, 112
Pet nutrition, 159
Pets, 131
Physical attractiveness, 8
Physiology of meditation, 43
Polio, 11
Popcorn, 165
"Pot bellies", 59
Pregnancy, 137
Preservatives, 3, 6, 10, 93, 108, 120, 123
Prevention, 1, 4, 9
Prevention Magazine, 36, 118
Psoriasis, xv
Psychiatrists/psychiatry, 1, 9, 51, 135
Psychosomatic diseases, 26, 39

Rancidity, 37, 109, 142, 143
Raw foods, 108
Reducing diets, 95

Religion, xiv, 19
Rice, 171
Rituals, 49
Rodale, J.I., 118
Rondiere, Pierre, 158
Roving, 92

Salad dressings, 112
Salt, 3, 35, 107, 117, 123, 142
Salt Awareness Chart, 119,
Saunas, 132
Scientific American, 43
Seasonings, 110
Self-esteem, 9, 30, 31, 37
Self-hypnosis, 56
Skin, 130
Skin disorders, 6
Small pox, 11
Smoking, xiv, 41, 141
Soup bases/stocks, 110
"Spare tires", 57
Spastic colon, 6
Spot meditation, 40, 54, 56
Steroids, 9
Stress, 9
Sugar, 3, 35, 107, 111, 114, 123
Sugar Awareness Chart, 117
Sugar Blues, 115, 138
Suggestions for supplements, 147
Sundaes, 166
Supplements (vitamins and minerals), 145
Sweeteners, 171
Swimming, 58, 90
Symptoms, 114

Tennis, 57
Theta brain wave level, 43, 52
Time limits, 13
Toxicity, vitamin, 155
Transcendental Meditation, 20, 49
Tubbingen, West Germany, 43
Tuberculosis, 11

Index

Ulcers, 6
University of California, 43

Vitamin supplements, 144
Vitamin toxicity, 155

Walking, 18, 36, 37, 91
Wallace, Robert Keith, 43
Wall Street Journal, The, 136, 141, 158
Washington Post, The, 141, 142
Water, 109, 141, 156, 171
"Weekend atheletes", 57
Weight reduction/dieting, 3, 58, 107
"What I Eat" Charts, 101
Wheat germ, 37
Whooping cough, 11
Williams, Roger, Ph.D., 97, 135
Workaholics, 29
Worksheets, 177
Wright, James Claude, 158

Yogis, 43
Yogurt, 36, 166, 169

Index to the Recipes

Anchovy Dip, 197
Avocado Dip, 197

Barbeque Sauce, 199
Bean Soup, 204
Bleu Cheese Salad Dressing or Dip, 197
Bread
  Basic Whole Wheat, 232
  No-knead Whole Wheat, 234
  Sourdough Applesauce Wheat, 233
Bread Starter, Whole Wheat Sourdough, 231
Brownies, Carob, 243

Cabbage Salad, 210

Carob Cake, 241
Carrot Cake, 239
Carrot Sandwich, Vegetarian, 195
Cereal, High Energy, 191
Cereal, Homemade, 191
Cheese Cake, 240
Chicken, Broiled Italian, 214
Chicken, Lemon Tarragon, 215
Chicken, Marengo Italiano, 216
Chicken, Breasts, Wine Savored, 215
Coconut Pie Shell, 238
Cookies, Carob Chip, 242
Cookies, Carob Chip-Oatmeal, 235
Corn, Roasted, 213
Crepes, Dessert, 241
Crepes, Savory, 219
Cucumber and Onion Salad, 211
Cucumbers and Onions, Marinated, Sweet and Sour, 209

Dill Dip, Elaine's, 196
Drink, Fruit Nutrition, 192
Drink, Nutrition, 192

Eggplant, Rice Casserole, 220
Eggplant, Stewed, 212
Egg Muffin, Healthy, 188
Eggs, Scrambled, 188

Fruit, Frozen Delight, 242
Fruit, Nut and Seed Candy, 237
Fudge, High Protein, 238
Fudge Sauce, New Health Hot, 234

Gazpacho, 201

Hamburgers, broiled, 230
Herbal Seasoning Salt, 200

Ketchup, Homemade, 200

Lamb, Roast with Herbs and Garlic, 217
Lasagna, Healthful, 225
Lentil Soup, Easy, 201

Index

Linguini, with White Clam Sauce, 224

Macaroni and Cheese, 229
Macaroni and Tuna Salad, 206
Mayonnaise, blender, 199
Mayonnaise and Yogurt Dressing, 210
McGuckin Special, 196
Mushrooms, Marinated, 28
Mushroom and Herb Salad, raw, 211

Omelet, basic, 189
Onion Dip, 198
Onion Soup, Carol and Luanne's, 202
Oysters, baked, 223

Pancakes, Whole Wheat, 190
Peaches, baked, 236
Peanut and Raisin Snack, 195
Peanut Butter, Homemade, 194
Peanut Butter and Jelly Sandwich, 194
Peanut Salad, Double Crunch, 206
Pie, Yogurt Cheese, 235
Pie Crust Mix, Standard Healthy, 239
Pie Crust, Whole Wheat, 236
Pineapple Coleslaw, 209
Pizza, 227
Pork Chops, Stuffed, 228
Potato Salad, 207
Potatoes, Oven, 213

Quiche Florentine, No-fail, 218

Roast, Creative Left-Over, 231
Roast, Tasty Pot, 229

Salmon Steaks Broiled with Herbs and Garlic, 222
Sausage, Homemade, 190
Scallops with White Wine and Herbs, 221

Soups
   Pat's Paradise Soup, 203
   Pea Soup, 203
   Hearty Vegetable, 205
Squash, Yellow Crooked Neck, 212
Swordfish, Steaks, broiled, 221

Tartar Sauce, 198
Tomato Juice Mix, 216
Trout, Stuffed, 224
Tuna Salad Sandwich, 193

Vegetables, lightly steamed, 214

Waldorf Salad Ambrosia, 208

Yogurt Shakes, 193
Yogurt Vinaigrette, 210

Breakfast Dishes
Cereal, High Energy, 191
Cereal, Homemade, 191
Drink, Nutrition, 192
Egg Muffin, Healthy, 188
Eggs, Scrambled, 188
Fruit Nutrition Drink, 192
Omelet, basic, 189
Pancakes, Whole Wheat, 190
Sausage, homemade, 190
Yogurt Shakes, 193

Sandwiches
Carrot Sandwich, Vegetarian, 195
Peanut Butter and Jelly Sandwich, 194
Tuna Salad Sandwich, 193

Snacks
Fruit, Nut and Seed Candy, 237
McGuckin Special, 196
Peanut and Raisin Snack, 195

Index

Dips and Condiments
Anchovy Dip, 197
Avocado Dip, 197
Barbeque Sauce, 199
Bleu Cheese Salad Dressing or Dip, 197
Dill Dip, Elaine's, 196
Herbal Seasoning Salt, 200
Ketchup, homemade, 200
Mayonnaise, blender, 199
Onion Dip, 198
Tartar Sauce, 198

Soups
Bean Soup, 204
Gazpacho, 201
Lentil Soup, Easy, 201
Onion Soup, Carol and Luanne's, 202
Pat's Paradise Soup, 203
Pea Soup, 203
Vegetable Soup, Healthy, 205

Salads
Macaroni and Tuna Salad, 206
Peanut Salad, Double Crunch, 206
Potato Salad, 207
Waldorf Salad Ambrosia, 208

Vetetables
Cabbage Salad, 210
Corn, roasted, 213
Cucumber and Onion Salad, 211
Cucumbers and Onions, Sweet and Sour Marinated, 209
Eggplant, stewed, 212
Mushroom and Herb Salad, raw, 211
Mushrooms, Marinated, 208
Pineapple Coleslaw, 209
Potatoes, Oven, 213
Squash, Yellow Crook Necked, 212
Vegetables, Lightly Steamed, 214

Main Dishes
Chicken, Broiled Italian, 214
Chicken, Lemon Tarragon, 215
Chicken, Marengo Italiano, 216
Chicken Breasts, Wine-Savored, 215
Crepes, Savory, 219
Eggplant Rice Casserole, 220
Hamburgers, broiled, 230
Lamb with Herbs and Garlic, Roast, 217
Lasagna, Healthful, 225
Linguini, with White Clam Sauce, 224
Macaroni and Cheese, 229
Oysters, baked, 223
Pizza, 227
Pot Roast, Tasty, 229
Quiche Florentine, No-Fail, 218
Roast, Creative Left-Over, 231
Salmon Steaks Broiled with Herbs and Garlic, 222
Scallops with White Wine and Herbs, 221
Swordfish Steaks, Broiled, 221
Trout, Stuffed, 224

Breads
Whole Wheat, No-Knead, 234
Sourdough Applesauce, 233
Whole Wheat, Basic, 232
Bread Starter, Whole Wheat Sourdough, 231

Desserts
Baked Peaches, 236
Carob Brownies, 243
Carob Cake, 239
Carob Chip Cookies, 242
Carob Chip-Oatmeal Cookies, 235
Carrot Cake , 239
Cheese Cake, 240
Coconut Pie Shell, 238
Dessert Crepes, 241
Frozen Fruit Delight, 242
Fruit, Nut and Seed Candy, 237
Fudge, High Protein, 238
Hot Fudge Sauce, 234

Index

Pie Crust Mix, Standard Healthy, 239
Pie Crust, Whole Wheat, 236
Yogurt Cheese Pie, 235

Party Dishes
Bar-B-Q Beef, 245
Chicken Salad, Hot, 246
Clam Squares, Hot, 244
Kidney Bean Salad with Cheese and
 Apples, 246
Variation Fruit Salad, 247